# How To Live
# While Loving A Manic Depressive

By Lynn Bradley

Library of Congress
Cataloging of Publication Division
101 Independence Ave, S.E.
Washington, D. C. 20540-4320


Library of Congress Cataloging-in-Publication Data

Bradley, Lynn.

Manic depression: how to live while loving a manic depressive / by
    Lynn Bradley
                            p. cm.
ISBN 1-885373-28-7 (softcover)
        1. Manic-depressive illness--Patients. 2. Depression, Mental. I.
    Title.
                    RC516 .B73 2000
                    616.89'5--dc21
                    00-009715               ⁄

Printed in the United States of America

# Acknowledgements

From the moment I met Bob, I knew he was the man I would spend the rest of my life with. He loved children; he laughed a lot; he made me laugh. More importantly, we had the same moral values and both expected our marriage to be a permanent commitment. When manic-depression became stronger than either of us, before we knew what was wrong with him, I would cry and mentally chant, "Where is my Bob?" Without my Bob, there would be no book. Throughout his struggle to maintain his mental health, he has consistently encouraged my writing. I thank him for the life we've shared, the rough and the smooth, the rich and the poor, and for agreeing to allow me the privilege of sharing our experience with you. Thanks, honey.

I also thank my critique group for listening to chapters repeatedly until I got them right. They were and are invaluable in helping me see how a person unfamiliar with manic-depression responds. Thanks, guys.

I also want to thank Donald E. Hauser, M.D. His diagnosis and treatment have saved Bob's life, I have no doubt, but his caring means as much to me as it does to Bob. He is a compassionate man and wise beyond his years. In the art of diagnosing Bipolar Illness, he is a genius. Over the years, we have recommended him to many friends, without hesitation. So, Dr. Don, thank you for all you have done for us.

May God bless you all

*Lynn Bradley.*

# Contents

# Foreword

by Donald E. Hauser, M.D.

The awareness of manic depressive illness has been around for centuries. It has been eloquently described in poetic and medical literature from Homer to Hippocrates. Aretaeus described both mania and melancholy as sharply as any modern observer. As we went into the dark ages, most of this knowledge was suppressed, and people suffering from manic depression were thought of as being possessed by demons, or even as witches. However, after the Renaissance, we seemed to rediscover the phenomena described ages earlier, and these people were treated by psychiatrists, and treated as the mentally ill. We now conceptualize this disease as an aberration of a DNA strand on a specific chromosome.

It was in 1896 that Emil Kraepelin actually coined the name *manic depressive insanity*. This later became manic depressive illness, and is now known as Bipolar Disorder, with various subtypes.

Over the years, there have been thousands of articles and books written on the etiology, diagnosis, and treatment of manic depressive illness. Very few have ever written on how people in society, non-mental health workers, feel about people with manic depressive illness.

How does a person deal with someone who is charming and charismatic, while also being unpredictable and impulsive? And at another time is melancholic and suicidal? How does the family of the manic depressive deal with these swings, while trying to maintain a stable environment with the remaining members of the family? How do friends and family help the person seek help when the symptoms of the disease encourage the person to shun help? How do all the people who are in contact with this person make sense of their own lives, while riding along on this emotional roller coaster?

Lynn Bradley attempts to answer these and other questions that are asked by those of us who are consistently around people with Bipolar Disorder. Who is more qualified to get us through the ropes of dealing with a manic depressive than someone who has lived with one for more than thirty years?

You will find this book educational, informative, and useful in regard to manic depressive illness and to mental illnesses in general. Books like this one, along with mental health support groups, such as DMDA (Depressive/Manic Depressive Association), are vital in de-stigmatizing mental illness. They also make us aware that the treatment of illnesses, such as Manic

Depressive Disorder, should be exactly as other "medical" illnesses in our society.

I recommend this book to anyone who has compassion or wants to have compassion for those who suffer from mental illness, and for their families that suffer with them.

*Donald E. Hauser, M.D.*
**The Hauser Clinic, Houston, Texas**

# A Note From Bob

My wife is the author of this fine text. My sole contributions were the bipolar illness I inherited from my father and my experience in recovery. Before she started, she talked with me because the book delves into my private world—my private world of insanity and my special quirks. I considered the readers and any possible consequences of my exposure for a millisecond and said, "Get after it!"

There have been questions by friends and family about our strange tendency to share our life and our problems. My feelings about this sharing can be described as being dragged through hell with my back broke. But if it can help one bipolar for one second to escape the pain I've known, then I would be willing to tell my life's story in living color on the Tonight Show.

I am a very fortunate mental patient. Without my wife, I wouldn't be alive. Without my children and friends, I would be huddled in a dark corner, contemplating my next suicide attempt.

For whatever reasons, I am a proud and independent man, which can be terminal for a manic-depressive like me. By some miracle, I've had hands help me tear down that barrier of independence. I have learned to ask for help and then accept it. If I have to give up my independence, but receive so much help, then I owe some form of contribution to others. This is my indirect contribution to ease the pain of other bipolars and those who love them.

This book has the normal human errors and weaknesses that literary work has contained since the mud tablets of Babylon, but there is one ingredient it doesn't lack. That is love. The love Lynn and I have for each other, the love our children and grandchildren have for us and the immense love our friends have demonstrated is on every page.

I hope you find a spark of hope in here that will enable you to try one more day with your bipolar and join Lynn and me as we trudge the road of happy destiny.

Love,
Bob

# Introduction

If you've ever loved a manic-depressive, someone diagnosed as having Bipolar Disorder, you took one of two courses: you ran away (emotionally or physically) as fast as you could, or you spent hours and hours trying to figure out how to control the person's moods. I believe I've found a third alternative.

My way of dealing with manic-depressive illness is, however, most practical if the patient is in full compliance with doctor's orders. Even if the person is a willing participant in the maintenance of his or her own mental health, the going won't be smooth.

What I hope to do is show you in an intensely personal way what I did, what works for me, and how it can help you. I am not a doctor and have no special training in this area. What I have is many years of experience. I have already made more mistakes than necessary. I've also discovered a few solutions.

Reading this book may make a difference in whether or not you stay in the relationship with the bipolar in your life.

If you are hopelessly in love and would quit loving the manic-depressive if you could, you are like me. I have been married to my manic-depressive for over thirty years, none of it dull, much of it exciting, all of it puzzling. Learning what causes his mood swings, what to do about it and what not to do about it has been helpful.

Learning what to do with me has saved our marriage.

I believe this book will be most helpful if you read straight through the first time, then go back and apply some of the exercises—as needed. Daily journaling is helpful for not only coping with a manic-depressive, but for coping with life in general. Since there are so many books and classes on journaling, I have not gone into the process here. You may want to check it out on your own.

I know that in the years to come, I will discover many more problems and solutions. This time I'll take notes and pass them on to you in my next book.

God bless you.

*Lynn*

# Contents

# Foreword

by Donald E. Hauser, M.D.

The awareness of manic depressive illness has been around for centuries. It has been eloquently described in poetic and medical literature from Homer to Hippocrates. Aretaeus described both mania and melancholy as sharply as any modern observer. As we went into the dark ages, most of this knowledge was suppressed, and people suffering from manic depression were thought of as being possessed by demons, or even as witches. However, after the Renaissance, we seemed to rediscover the phenomena described ages earlier, and these people were treated by psychiatrists, and treated as the mentally ill. We now conceptualize this disease as an aberration of a DNA strand on a specific chromosome.

It was in 1896 that Emil Kraepelin actually coined the name *manic depressive insanity*. This later became manic depressive illness, and is now known as Bipolar Disorder, with various subtypes.

Over the years, there have been thousands of articles and books written on the etiology, diagnosis, and treatment of manic depressive illness. Very few have ever written on how people in society, non-mental health workers, feel about people with manic depressive illness.

How does a person deal with someone who is charming and charismatic, while also being unpredictable and impulsive? And at another time is melancholic and suicidal? How does the family of the manic depressive deal with these swings, while trying to maintain a stable environment with the remaining members of the family? How do friends and family help the person seek help when the symptoms of the disease encourage the person to shun help? How do all the people who are in contact with this person make sense of their own lives, while riding along on this emotional roller coaster?

Lynn Bradley attempts to answer these and other questions that are asked by those of us who are consistently around people with Bipolar Disorder. Who is more qualified to get us through the ropes of dealing with a manic depressive than someone who has lived with one for more than thirty years?

You will find this book educational, informative, and useful in regard to manic depressive illness and to mental illnesses in general. Books like this one, along with mental health support groups, such as DMDA (Depressive/Manic Depressive Association), are vital in de-stigmatizing mental illness. They also make us aware that the treatment of illnesses, such as Manic Depressive Disorder, should be exactly as other "medical" illnesses in our society.

I recommend this book to anyone who has compassion or wants to have compassion for those who suffer from mental illness, and for their families that suffer with them.

*Donald E. Hauser, M.D.*
**The Hauser Clinic, Houston, Texas**

# A Note From Bob

My wife is the author of this fine text. My sole contributions were the bipolar illness I inherited from my father and my experience in recovery. Before she started, she talked with me because the book delves into my private world—my private world of insanity and my special quirks. I considered the readers and any possible consequences of my exposure for a millisecond and said, "Get after it!"

There have been questions by friends and family about our strange tendency to share our life and our problems. My feelings about this sharing can be described as being dragged through hell with my back broke. But if it can help one bipolar for one second to escape the pain I've known, then I would be willing to tell my life's story in living color on the Tonight Show.

I am a very fortunate mental patient. Without my wife, I wouldn't be alive. Without my children and friends, I would be huddled in a dark corner, contemplating my next suicide attempt.

For whatever reasons, I am a proud and independent man, which can be terminal for a manic-depressive like me. By some miracle, I've had hands help me tear down that barrier of independence. I have learned to ask for help and then accept it. If I have to give up my independence, but receive so much help, then I owe some form of contribution to others. This is my indirect contribution to ease the pain of other bipolars and those who love them.

This book has the normal human errors and weaknesses that literary work has contained since the mud tablets of Babylon, but there is one ingredient it doesn't lack. That is love. The love Lynn and I have for each other, the love our children and grandchildren have for us and the immense love our friends have demonstrated is on every page.

I hope you find a spark of hope in here that will enable you to try one more day with your bipolar and join Lynn and me as we trudge the road of happy destiny.

Love,

Bob

# Introduction

If you've ever loved a manic-depressive, someone diagnosed as having Bipolar Disorder, you took one of two courses: you ran away (emotionally or physically) as fast as you could, or you spent hours and hours trying to figure out how to control the person's moods. I believe I've found a third alternative.

My way of dealing with manic-depressive illness is, however, most practical if the patient is in full compliance with doctor's orders. Even if the person is a willing participant in the maintenance of his or her own mental health, the going won't be smooth.

What I hope to do is show you in an intensely personal way what I did, what works for me, and how it can help you. I am not a doctor and have no special training in this area. What I have is many years of experience. I have already made more mistakes than necessary. I've also discovered a few solutions.

Reading this book may make a difference in whether or not you stay in the relationship with the bipolar in your life.

If you are hopelessly in love and would quit loving the manic-depressive if you could, you are like me. I have been married to my manic-depressive for over thirty years, none of it dull, much of it exciting, all of it puzzling. Learning what causes his mood swings, what to do about it and what not to do about it has been helpful.

Learning what to do with me has saved our marriage.

I believe this book will be most helpful if you read straight through the first time, then go back and apply some of the exercises—as needed. Daily journaling is helpful for not only coping with a manic-depressive, but for coping with life in general. Since there are so many books and classes on journaling, I have not gone into the process here. You may want to check it out on your own.

I know that in the years to come, I will discover many more problems and solutions. This time I'll take notes and pass them on to you in my next book.

*God bless you.*

*Lynn*

# How To Live
# While Loving a Manic-Depressive

by Lynn Bradley

*The beginning of wisdom is to call things by their right name*
*—Chinese Proverb*

Why doesn't he even try to control his temper? Why can't he change for my sake? What mood will he be in when I get home? What am I doing wrong? These are only a few of the questions I asked myself over and over.

I hated him.

I hated me.

I hated my life.

It was hard for me to understand why I'd ever married my husband. Bob had been verbally abusive, made and lost several fortunes and had a sex drive and technique that... oh, yeah. Now I remember why I married him.

Old enough to know better, but too young to care, I began dating Bob when he was still Bobby, a golden-haired, made-me-laugh kind of guy with sparkling blue eyes and a lopsided grin hardly any female, from three to ninety-three, could resist.

Whenever I remembered our courtship and our early years of marriage, I seldom looked at all the evictions, overdrawn bank accounts, frequent moves and job changes. I focused instead on him rolling on the floor, laughing with our children, dancing me around in the kitchen, and long, hand-in-hand walks on the beach, him sharing his wonderful goals and dreams for our future.

But there I was in the lobby of Memorial Southwest Hospital in Houston, Texas, hating my life and hating him. Most of all I was afraid I'd have to take home an over-medicated zombie incapable of the rudimentary requirements for daily life. I knew I couldn't cope; I couldn't be responsible for *everything*.

Today, ten years later, I realize I was as sick as he was, but in a different way with a different "illness." My illness was not inherited; it was acquired by long-term exposure to his. Donald E. Hauser, M.D., diagnosed Bob as having manic-depression.

I'm not manic-depressive, but I *am* a manic-depressive magnet. If there's a manic-depressive within a hundred miles of me, I'll take out my radar and zero in on him or her. They'll become fast friends or weird incidents, but I'll find them. Just call me Magnet.

But I am not alone. I am not sure if we magnets find the bipolars or if they find us, but we do tend to hook up on a regular basis.

One woman I interviewed, Marian, told me about dissolving her long friendship with Judy, a manic-depressive. Losing the friendship was painful for Marian. Through tears, she said, "We'd had some really good times together. Then one time when we had planned a trip to Galveston, she called about thirty minutes before I expected her to pick me up. She said she didn't feel like doing the beach. She was going to a movie with some guy."

"Hadn't she done that sort of thing before?" I asked.

"Sure, but that was the last straw. I don't have to keep letting her screw up my plans. Real friends don't do what she did."

The next time I saw Marian she introduced me to her new friend and running-buddy, Wendy. I later learned that the vivacious Wendy with the huge smile was also manic-depressive.

I rest my case.

Learning to call things by their right name is a true blessing. It frees me to get on with finding a solution, a coping strategy. I don't like or dislike being called handicapped or a cripple, and since 1993 lupus has affected my ankle joints and caused me to walk funny when I walk, and ride in a wheelchair when I don't. I had to accept the fact and the condition of being crippled before I could submit

3

to the wheelchair on an as-needed basis without feeling sorry for myself.

Facts are facts, and I yam what I yam. Knowing I'm a manic-depressive magnet, I wasn't surprised one afternoon while I was taking an outdoors lunch break from my office job in a hospital building atrium. I sat with three other women on the picnic benches near the back door. A man bustled from the building and hurried past us. About ten feet beyond our table, he whirled around and walked straight back to me. I'd never seen the guy in my life.

He said, "I just got out of this hospital. I was on the tenth floor (the psychiatric floor) and they decided I'm manic-depressive. Can you believe that?" He leaned toward me, obviously expecting an answer.

I nodded and assured him I not only believed it, I could confirm it.

Just what is manic-depressive or bipolar disorder and how do I radar in on them? How do they find me? I may never know, but they truly do.

The more important question is how do I live with and love a manic-depressive and hang on to my own sanity? And why? Maybe I need the enthusiasm and unexpected excitement Bob brings into our lives. Maybe he needs the way I laugh at his jokes. I believe the answer lies in that great line from the film "Rocky," the original: We fill gaps.

Before I answer the "how" question, I want to establish a definition of manic-depressive, or manic-depressive disease, also know as bipolar disorder. (The terms will be used interchangeably throughout this book.)

You may have noticed that the jargon of psychiatry has slipped into our vocabularies to such a degree that most of us have heard many labels or diagnoses of mental illnesses and disorders. But don't we, unless we are affected, have only a vague idea of their true meaning?

Current myths lead us to believe some rather bizarre and distorted half-truths concerning all mental illnesses and basically lump them together in a "Cuckoo's Nest." One rampant idea is that anyone experiencing mood swings is probably manic-depressive. I did not realize how prevalent this attitude is until a podiatrist said to me, "Oh, we're all a little manic-depressive from time to time, don't you think?"

This is not true. Yet, here was an educated man, a doctor, making a blanket statement about a medical condition totally out of his area of expertise. People within hearing distance may well have filed that statement away, making their understanding of manic-depression not only inadequate, but minimizing the condition and relegating it to the position of other universal maladies. "We all get a cold from time to time, don't you think?"

Of course, everyone does have ups and downs. For the non-bipolars, they stay within "normal" limits. A manic-depressive's reactions to life are divided into elation—everything's going my way; and despair—nothing ever goes my way. When the manic-depressive in my life reaches the latter stage, I mentally refer to it as playing End-of-the-World. I know his perception of life is going to change; he doesn't.

Before Bob's diagnosis in 1987, I had been diagnosed with lupus, an auto-immune dysfunction sometimes called the disease of a thousand faces. I get clinically depressed, too. But my depression is much less severe, rarely contains suicidal ideation and is easily controlled with medication. Because of my illness, I do understand the down side of his.

Whenever I'm depressed, I truly believe I've *always* felt exactly the way I feel at the time. Unlike the *emotion* depression, the *illness* depression cycles regardless of external circumstances, although external conditions may trigger or exacerbate onset.

As for the emotion depression, everyone experiences it from time to time in reaction to life. In most instances, it is expected and normal: loss of a loved one through death or divorce, loss of a job, etc. In less painful situations we may feel a little blue because we're bored or lonely so we say we're depressed. Maybe we even cry. Then external circumstances change and our mood changes. We get a long worked-for promotion, find the perfect blouse on sale, get a phone call from a friend and feel so excited we're sure we merely misunderstood what was out of sorts. Or we declare, "Thank goodness, that mood passed."

People with bipolar disorder often describe their depression as a descending black fog. When Winston Churchill suffered from depression, he announced, "— the black dog has come to visit."

Some affected people hear a voice in the fog that tells them the only way to escape their terrible dilemma is suicide. Their suicidal ideation often includes elaborate plans for the scene where they'll be found and their funeral service with pallbearers and mourners named.

The flip-side of bipolar illness is *mania*. A so-called normal manic reaction to life could come as a spontaneous purchase, a sudden delight in a spring day, a burst of energy or song. These reactions do not indicate a true mania.

A manic episode can often cause bipolars to appear very enthusiastic, confident and charming. It also accelerates to delusions of grandiosity and a firm belief that they have the answers to the world's problems and can fly if need be. Additionally, most believe they are invincible. Some claim to be on a first-name basis with God or the Spirit of the Universe and may hallucinate.

If you're living with or in love with someone either suspected of having manic-depressive disease or who has been diagnosed with bipolar disorder, you may have become a victim of their illness. If you are determined to stay close to that person, you may be a magnet. You may also be very compassionate or very naïve.

In maintaining the relationship you will discover, as I have, that accepted truths no longer apply. For example: If doing the same thing and *expecting* different results is insanity, what is it when we do the same thing and *get* different results?

Whatever it is, it makes us crazy—if we don't understand what changed the manic-depressive's thinking and caused such unexpected results.

To illustrate what happens when we become victims of their illness, let me tell you about Sue. In looking back over her marriage of twelve years, she swears that in the early years she had to wait until Tom woke up to see what mood she was in. Sue, like many of us, tolerated her husband's temper outbursts and depression withdrawals in exchange for the excitement his hypomania brought into her life.

In his book, *Feeling Good* (Signet 1980), David D. Burns, MD, describes manic-depression:

> The symptoms include an abnormally elated or irritable mood that persists for at least two days and is not caused by drugs or alcohol. The manic patient's behavior is characterized by impulsive actions which reflect poor judgment (such as irresponsible, excessive spending) along with a grandiose sense of self-confidence. Mania is accompanied by increased sexual or aggressive activity; hyperactive, continuous body movements;

racing thoughts, nonstop, excited talking; and a decreased need to sleep. Manic individuals have the delusion that they are extraordinarily powerful and brilliant, and often insist they are on the verge of some philosophical or scientific breakthrough or lucrative money-making scheme.

Notice his description declares this abnormality is *not* caused by drugs or alcohol, although according to *Handbook of Drug Therapy in Psychiatry,* by Jerrold G. Bernstein: "There is a high correlation between manic episodes and the tendency to consume excessive quantities of alcohol." This of course, may lead to the disease of alcoholism or chemical dependency.

While I don't want to get into a "chicken or egg" discussion, I do want to stress that treatment for alcoholism or chemical dependency, when needed, will benefit the manic-depressive, but will not relieve the mental illness of the disease.

Bipolar disorder is a physical dysfunction in which the biological ingredients required to make rational decisions and exhibit appropriate moods are not present in the affected person's brain. Treatment of chemical dependency, alcoholism or drug addiction is often unsuccessful for manic-depressives unless their brain disease is treated simultaneously.

While the foregoing description of bipolar disorder is certainly not that of a healthy individual's reaction to life, it is equally important to recognize that loving these all-or-nothing people isn't exactly normal, either. It can cause a person to behave as irrationally as a bipolar. Anxiety, frustration, anger, fear, and guilt impair our mental and emotional health. We begin to doubt our own sense of reality. We wonder if we can stand our life another minute—another second. We never know what we will come home to. We never know if the meal we serve will be praised or thrown against the wall.

We also know that if we hear a clever retort that we wish we'd said, quite probably some manic-depressive has already said it.

For years I tried to make sense out of Bob's decisions whether it was to buy a new car, (mine needs new tires—must be time to get a new one), or move (I can't make the rent here and we're getting evicted, so let's rent this more expensive place), or change jobs (I've never made a living in the business I left three years ago, so I think I should try it one more time).

All of those decisions and many others of the same type, made more than once, actually made sense at the time—even to me. Manic-depressives can be very convincing.

There were also times when his decisions didn't make sense. I believed him when he told me I was stupid or crazy and didn't understand how the world worked. Most manic-depressives can be *extremely* convincing.

While I tried to make sense out of my life, he kept grinning, dancing and laughing until I believed he was going to make me wonderfully happy—someday. He would get us there quicker if only I would quit trying to put limits on him. He was sure we would soon be millionaires, visit exotic places and wear nothing but designer clothes.

Even when I knew his ideas were distorted, I sometimes went along, not wanting to spoil his great fun and enthusiasm. I agreed to the BMW and Trans Am we couldn't afford; I committed to future fun I knew we'd never experience. I began to wonder if I weren't making molehills out of his beautiful mountains when I attempted to resist his brilliance. Was I losing my mind? I wondered.

Then, unfortunately, we did exactly that—became millionaires, visited exotic places and wore designer clothes. We also lived on two acres in a large house with swimming pool, hot tub, greenhouse, garage apartment, maids, barn, one calf, four sheep, umpteen chickens that laid green eggs, and I have no idea how many rabbits. We even had a pear tree.

I said "unfortunately" because when we reached that financial state, I became convinced he'd been right all along and I had been uninformed, uneducated and had shown no faith in his ability to provide for us.

For a few years, all seemed to be falling into place. We gave our adult children lavish gifts—like houses or condos and cars. We traveled to Europe a few times, the Caribbean, Mexico—anywhere my little old heart desired.

As much fun as it all was, I had this "waiting for the other shoe to drop" feeling. In spite of all the money Bob made, it was never enough. I had no idea that three years or so down the road we'd be plunged into bankruptcy. Yet, it was not really all that surprising. We both knew something was wrong with Bob. We didn't know what.

He kept "coming down with something." He would wake up, especially on Monday mornings, with an atrocious headache, say he felt like he was coming down with the flu or a virus, crawl back into bed and stay there for one to four days, or a week or two. His internal medicine doctor could find nothing wrong.

During that siege of medical mysteries, (two years prior to his diagnosis), I saw a television program about manic-depression and suggested to our doctor at that time that the information sounded a lot like Bob. The doctor said, "Oh, I don't think so. I've never seen Bob down or even the least bit depressed."

Of course he hadn't. No one had ever seen Bob depressed except me—and I didn't know I was looking at depression when it filled the house with its darkness. If Bob ever left the house when he was depressed, which was rare, he exhibited rage more than anything else. I had no idea his ill temper was a result of his disease.

As a matter of fact, there was practically nothing I knew except what I'd seen on television. The show I remember led me to believe my husband would end up in a halfway house for the mentally incompetent, and I'd end up living with relatives or in a psychiatric facility trying to figure out what I'd done wrong. Fortunately, it never came to that.

Bipolar disorder is not contagious. Ulcers are not contagious, either, but living with a manic-depressive may give you one. Yes, I know there is a type of ulcer that is caused by a virus, and another kind caused by taking aspirin-type medications that irritate stomach lining. The stress-induced type, however... well, this isn't a book about ulcer disease. Suffice it to say, if I had to identify manic-depressives as ulcer types or ulcer-carrier types, I'd have to call them carriers. But it's not intentional.

Hardly anything they do is intentional. Just as my intentions and actions sometimes don't match up, which confuses me, their actions, words, accusations and outbursts are often as mysterious to them as they are to us. I want to point out some important facts about this:

1. It is *my* reactions that make me crazy—not his.

2. If I didn't react so quickly, maybe I could stop reacting and act.

3.  Whenever I expect him to behave in a pre-
    dictable manner, I *am* crazy.

One reason I react so strongly to anything he does that seems even a little weird is that I keep expecting him to behave in a manner I call "normal." He does perform such wonderful normal acts, sometimes for days. During that time, I delude myself into believing he has been somehow magically cured and will never again do or say anything I consider "crazy."

I believe another reason I react so quickly and so strongly is that his mania is my addiction. I get my lift, my "fix," or my excitement by being with him when he's even slightly manic (*hypomanic*). That fun stage is what attracted me to him in the first place. It's what makes him such a good salesman, such an excellent conversationalist, or life of the party when there is no party. He talks to everyone he comes across—in elevators, grocery stores, places he's never been before. Everyone he acknowledges seems happier for it. I latch onto his arm and beam as if I'd built him myself.

When his psychiatrist, Dr. Hauser, first talked to me about Bob's condition, he told me there are several consistently, though not required, observable symptoms most manic-depressives present: incomplete college education, good (if somewhat sporadic) salesman or very good with people in general, and have usually had multiple marriages or relationships. Our long-lasting marriage almost fooled him into a misdiagnosis.

It is often the second to fifth spouse who shows up at a psychiatric hospital, trying to do better than any previous spouse at understanding and helping (or controlling) the poor misunderstood manic-depressive.

There are several ways I tried to control Bob before we knew what was wrong with him. If he got quiet, angry or wouldn't get out of bed, I secretly telephoned friends and invited them over. I knew he "came out of his funk" around other people, which I deeply resented. After all, if he loved me as much as he claimed, why wouldn't he perk up for me?

Whenever he left home in a foul mood, I'd spend the day cleaning. In a warped sense of my importance to his moods, I'd decided my lack of housekeeping had set him off that morning. Then after scrubbing everything nailed down and laundering anything that wasn't, I'd cook a favorite meal and greet him with a tentative smile when he returned.

If I didn't get my desired response, although sometimes I did, I'd go into the bathroom and cry. When my ploy seemed to work, I reassured myself that now I had a handle on how to manage his moods, only to be thrown off the next time it didn't work.

I tried other methods of controlling him, which sometimes worked and sometimes didn't. Mostly, I felt crazy, disoriented, off-balance and out of tune. It is this sickness within the minds and emotions of spouses and friends who stick with the manic-depressives that most often gets no treatment at all.

Knowing that someone you care about is sick and what that entails is beneficial. Knowing what you can do to help a person with bipolar disorder stay on a medication regime is admirable. Knowing when to contact his doctor, what signs indicate he needs attention, when to leave him alone... all that is important. But knowing what to do with *your* anger, fear, anxiety and frustration is what this book is all about.

If you love a manic-depressive, you know exactly what I mean.

# Chapter 2

*"It's not my fault"*

—*Homer Simpson*

At age thirteen, I stomped off, angry that Daddy wouldn't let me go to the movie with my friends. I kicked my little brother's toy xylophone the length of the hall. Daddy dashed to see if I had been hurt. He was sure I'd fallen.

"Honey, are you all right?"

Dripping pure innocence, I said, "Yeah, I guess so, but if it's broken, it's not my fault. He shouldn't have left it in the hall."

It worked. It always worked. If I blamed someone else, I didn't get into trouble. Whenever anything happened that could possibly cause me a problem, I had three younger siblings to blame.

In marriage, I found the same solution to avoiding problems: blame anyone; accept responsibility for nothing.

Of course, I didn't realize what I was doing. I truly believed it should be clear to everyone that it (whatever *it* was that day) wasn't my fault. I believed everything in my life that felt wrong, out of step with the world, or particularly burdensome was Bob's fault. The fact that I loved him, married him, stayed married to him, was my only contribution to my troubles.

I was certain if he would only... (and here the list goes on like that pink bunny), then our life would change, and I'd be "happily ever after."

My favorite conversation topics always included long-suffering tales of our latest woes. One afternoon while grocery shopping I encountered a woman I hadn't seen in several months. She made a terrible mistake when she opened her mouth to greet me. She asked how I was doing.

I promptly went into our latest travails, complete with agonizing groans, disgusted smirks, and unspoken pleas for sympathy.

Loretta backed up her cart and overtly eyed me from hairdo to sandals. She shook her head as if she couldn't believe what she'd observed. I was positive she intended to say she wondered how I managed. Instead, she said, "Damn, Lynn, you look terrific in that martyr cloak!"

Slightly puffed up with indignation, I said, "I am not a martyr. You asked how I'm doing and I told you."

She grinned. "No, sweetie, you told me how you think Bob is doing."

I don't know that anyone else would have had the nerve to tell me the truth like that. I'm grateful for her and all the Lorettas in my life. What surprises me most, however, is that I knew she was right. When I mentally reviewed what I'd told her, I realized almost every sentence had begun with "Bob said, or Bob did, or Bob didn't."

I had no idea how I was doing.

I began to examine my life. My life, which means my thoughts and my actions, had to change or I'd be forever a martyr and forever miserable.

I'd made assumptions and poor choices that had nothing to do with Bob. My consistent choices had been to play victim and seek sympathy. I decided the next time anyone asked me how I was doing, I'd pretend Bob didn't exist. I'd stick to my own thoughts and actions. It turned out to be far more difficult than I'd anticipated.

I made many false starts. "I'm a little tired. Bob—" then I'd start over. "I'm a little tired. I read into the wee hours, and had a hard time getting up this morning."

After that, if they asked how Bob was doing, I suggested they give him a call, and said that he'd probably like to hear from them.

I wish I could say I am "cured" and all my decisions and choices are good now, but that is not the case. Blaming Bob is still my first choice when anything goes wrong.

While Bob made many poor choices on his own, (primarily because of his illness, but sometimes because of inexperience), if his choice brought disaster, I was quick to remind him it was his fault we got into trouble. I proclaimed him king of the manor, but with my sneaky, underhanded ways, I usually "led" him to making the decision I wanted him to make, still claiming it wasn't my fault.

If I overtly make decisions, then I have to be responsible. If he makes all decisions, any misery I suffer is definitely his fault.

The biggest problem with my method is the number I do on myself to live with what I've done. I thought of myself as a victim. A poor, helpless victim. And, yes, a martyr.

Being a victim is hard work. It is also a do-it-yourself project. By that, I mean unless you are truly victimized by someone evil, no one is out to get you. The only way to become a victim is to set yourself up.

I'm sure there are many ways to do this, but I've found and perfected a few that always worked for me. The price, in self-esteem, can get a little steep, but you get what you pay for. I can back myself into a corner where the only explanation I (or anyone who will listen to me) can logically come up with is "he did it to me again."

If it hadn't been for Loretta, I don't know if I'd have ever seen that truth. I was really good at self-deception and placing blame!

Here's how it goes: First, I select any one of his quirks or petty, annoying habits. Then I set about to "help him" change it.

One example is the way he stacks the dishes in the sink. He's always done it the same way. Whichever hand reaches the sink first deposits the first dish. Sensible, I suppose, except that the hand holding his drinking glass always gets there first. In it goes. The plate or bowl goes next, precariously balanced on top. If there's a bowl *and* a plate, the bowl goes between the glass and plate. A wonderfully creative tower, but one of my pet peeves developed over years of turning on the water and having it splash onto the counter or down the front of my clothes.

Of course, I can see how the dishes are stacked and I know where the water will go, but I can't feel sorry for myself if I don't get wet.

My next step is to gently tell him exactly how much his creative building annoys me. Which loosely translated means: *Don't you dare do that again.* But of course, he does. So I smile to myself and remember he's only acting out of habit and didn't mean to annoy me. I carefully re-stack the dishes in their "proper" order, feeling very pleased with my calm, non-visible reaction and am hopeful he will take note of the proper arrangement.

I usually stay in this mode for several days, through several episodes of improper stacking. But soon afterward comes my fall to victimization. I walk into the kitchen, see his "tower," turn on the tap, get wet and freak.

Poor me. I have to live with this crazy man who cannot fathom the simple rules for stacking dishes. Oh, woe is me!

I usually feel like throwing the dishes at him, but I only re-stack them, (with and without heavy sighs), convinced I am doomed to suffer at his hands throughout eternity.

Now, this all sounds too funny. How could anyone get so upset over how the dishes are stacked? Hey, there are a bunch of women out there who would love to have their husbands carry the dishes to the sink. They'd be delighted to find dish-towers.

So what. I have to put up with his inane towers because he's a poor mental patient and can't be the man I thought I married, a fun-loving manic who made me feel as if dish-towers were not only normal, but much preferred.

And that's only one example of setting myself up. My victimization always happens when I expect him to be someone he never was and can never be.

Another example of how I try to "help" him may make more sense than the way he stacks dishes in the sink, but you get the idea.

Of course, he neither requires nor desires my help, but I'm sure I know what he needs. (I throw in the mind reading for free, therefore, I *know* what he needs.)

I once decided he needed help placing our suitcases in the trunk of the car. We were headed for a fun weekend. In my mind, I merely "suggested" the smaller case would fit behind the spare tire. From his outburst, you would have thought I'd assaulted him. The problem wasn't what I said; it was how I said it, according to him.

I know he's right. In spite of my good intentions, I have a tendency to sound like a scolding big sister. What happened was my faith in his ability to do *anything* was shattered by his diagnosis. I judged everything he did against my conceptions of "normal" and "sane." I reached the point where I didn't believe he could do anything without my help. The first time, after he got out of the hospital, he wanted to go out alone I had a hard time letting him leave the house without me.

He'd spent most of his life taking care of himself. It didn't matter that my perception of his abilities had changed, and I no longer trusted his judgment. Instead of asking what he thought or discussing a subject, I monitored him. It was as if I were taking his temperature every ten minutes. One tenth of a degree in any direction and I stepped in to take over.

All I wanted to do was help.

When my help was rejected or ridiculed, I became righteously indignant, puffed myself up. I often declared that if my assistance was unappreciated, just see if I ever try to help again! And I'd think, *How can you treat me that way, after all I've done for you? Oh, poor pitiful me.*

I let him know I think I've been mistreated, though. I do it with body language, cabinet-door slamming, silence, anything he can't actually confront. If he comments on my mood, I tell him it has nothing to do with him. But while I'm telling him that, I believe it has everything to do with him. After all, it's not my fault.

So I bravely hold up my head and tell friends, "Oh, yes, Bob's taking his medication, but that doesn't fix everything. He still has his moments."

Internally, I hear a friend say, "She's such a strong woman. I don't see how she does it."

Sometimes, I hear, "She's such a strong woman. I don't see *why* she does it."

It gets back to that Magnet thing. I have a lot of manic-depressive friends. I forgive their shortcomings and character flaws. I'm Mother Teresa and Gandhi, and I want them to know it. I am so-o-o understanding. I can be stood up approximately 4.3 times, ignored 3.1 times, and I'll still call them my friends. If they go too far by .1 or more, I cry and wonder what I did wrong. Then I get mad. Then I forget I ever knew them. After all, I worked at our friendship and it's their fault we don't go to lunch anymore. I think it's their fault. I believe it's their fault.

Because I found it so easy to feel sorry for myself, I had a lot of dark secrets. They were humiliating and confusing. I was sure anyone sane would have me locked up for my own protection.

Secret No. 1: I had been called every vile name possible and accused of horrendous acts. No one in his right mind would put up with the verbal abuse I experienced and stayed married to the abuser. Was I as weak as the physically abused women I knew?

This "attack" mode is common in manic-depressives, with and without any basis in fact. It is only another way for them to run off anyone who cares about them—then they'll be truly alone and can commit suicide with a clear conscience. It will prove no one loves them. Depression can be very deadly.

Now I understand his tirades are a result of manic-depression, not necessarily anything I've done recently or in the past. He can't run me off. I also know telling him to stop is about as effective as telling someone with a virus to quit having diarrhea.

That secret and others encouraged me to blame him for everything I did that went against any basic principles. I felt so ashamed that I "took it" and never stood up for myself. Yet, with all my moaning and groaning to everyone who would listen, I never told anyone I *chose* to do what I did in order to keep peace at any price. And to stay married—for better or for worse. If I'd done anything differently, I'd have to admit my circumstances were my fault. And if it's not my fault, whose fault is it?

That question reminds me of another. If you show up at the hospital with a broken leg, does it really matter if you broke it by slipping on a banana peel or falling off a ladder? The admitting staff may ask, but no, of course it doesn't really matter. What matters is doing what has to be done to fix it.

Therein lies the real question. How do I quit blaming, shaming and accusing my manic-depressive of causing my problems? It's just so easy to blame him; he's the one with the mental problem. Right?

And just how crazy do I have to be to relinquish my freedom of choice? I stayed exactly that crazy for a long time. I was desperate to prevent the world from seeing the mistakes I'd made, and the ones I knew I'd make in the future. I didn't want to be a victim. It was all very perplexing.

Today, I am no longer a victim. The question: How did I change?

1. I had to recognize and accept that my problems are a result of my decisions. They *are* my fault. Not in the sense that I deliberately set myself up to cause my discomfort, but in the sense that I am the only one who can do anything change me.

2. I had to develop a plan and follow it. I did. This doesn't mean I no longer have problems, or even that I no longer have any of those same problems. It means I am no longer victimized by the problems that once dominated my life.

What, exactly, are my problems and how do I recognize them? That's where my "red flags" come in.

I spent several months watching my reactions and taking notes. Certain circumstances seemed to always lead to a red flag. At other times, red flags just popped up from some parallel universe where every emotion is labeled and all my active emotions are red flags.

One of the first flags to flip into view comes when my body tips me off or my actions change. Anytime I become aware of any one flag on the list, I probably need to step back and survey my attitude. If I see two or more flags on the same day, I'd better take positive action.

Other lists are scattered throughout this book, but here is the first Red Flag list.

## Red Flag List

1. Folding my arms across my chest

2. Cocking my hands on my hips

3. Slumping

4. Turning my back on him

5. Slamming doors

6. Driving too fast

7. Raising my voice

8. Clenching my jaw or my fists

9. Jerking, yanking or cursing anything

10. Complaining about him to others

When any of these flags appear and I don't take positive action quickly, I do something really stupid. Then I have to apologize, repair or replace.

I found a solution.

# Chapter 3

*Perplexity is the beginning of knowledge*
                                    —*Kahlil Gibran*

As the days unfolded after Bob's discharge from the hospital, it seemed as if I had more questions and fewer answers. I searched for solutions to carry me through his episodes, or any of his behaviors I thought suspect. Dr. Hauser loaned me several books, which I read very slowly. Being medical texts, it took heavy doses of concentration to digest the material—something I wasn't used to.

In the meantime, I found myself projecting, anticipating and dreading the coming days, months and years. I cried a lot. I felt powerless and hopeless. I wanted to run away. The man I depended upon was mentally ill. I knew I could never handle being the strong one in the family.

I went to my daughter's house, crying, and said, "I don't know what I'm going to do. I'm going to have to take care of everything!"

In her very practical way, she said, "Get real, Mother. You've been taking care of everything all your life."

When I thought about it, I knew she was right. Whenever we moved, which was often, I found the new place, contacted the utility companies and made all the arrangements to relocate the family. I also took care of everything else, except earning an income. For years I had supplemented his income doing everything from baby-sitting and sewing to working for a temporary agency.

Still, didn't believe I could cope.

I slipped slowly into clinical depression, not just a normal reaction to this new twist in my life. This change in my mood was a condition I neither recognized nor accepted, which stirred up a raging brain. I blamed Bob for my emotional state, my fears, my lupus, my life. I cried over nothing and everything. My eating pattern changed from a healthy diet to constant snacking on anything containing fat and sugar. I gained thirty pounds, felt too tired to exercise (even knowing that exercising would give me more energy), and roamed the house at night because I couldn't sleep. Other times I stayed in bed most of the day.

And always, I watched Bob for signs of encroaching insanity, fearful he'd do in himself. At the same time, I wished he'd get on with it if he were going to do it so I'd still be young enough to get over it and get on with my life. It wasn't that I wanted him dead; I wanted the problem to go away. His suicide looked like a solution for my problems.

My attitude toward him, my opinion of myself, and my constant fluctuations between love and hate—for him and for me—became very perplexing. Whatever was happening in my head, I didn't like it.

I read the list of symptoms published by National Alliance for Mental Health, but ignored the fact that any applied to me. All I looked for was proof that Bob was crazy and I wasn't.

Without being inside his head, there was no way for me to know what he was feeling or thinking. I kept reading, hoping I would find the magic key to fix him.

I learned that depression has always been evident in mankind. One of the earliest commentaries shows the disorder has not changed in more than 1,800 years.

In about 200 A. D. Plutarch described the feelings of a depressed man:

> He sits out of doors, wrapped in sack cloth or filthy rags. Ever and anon he rolls himself, naked, in the dirt confessing about this or that sin. He has eaten or drunk something wrong. He has gone some way or other which the divine being did not approve of.

Much more has been said and written, but that paragraph summed it up for me. Depressed persons feel that everything they have ever done was wrong. That's how I felt.

The depression experienced by spouses, friends and significant others of affected persons is not much different than the manic-depressive's mood dip into the lower sphere. It also responds to medication. Although medication doesn't solve everything, it gave me the opportunity to deal with my life more rationally. In addition to medication, I found other important steps to lessen the depth and duration of my depression.

The following list of symptoms will help you identify if depression has crept into your life. The American Psychiatric Association maintains that if any four of these symptoms persist for more than two weeks, you should seek professional help.

Usually after two days of symptoms, I *want* help—and so does Bob.

1) Noticeable change of appetite (weight loss when not dieting or unintentional and unwanted weight gain);

2) Noticeable change in sleeping pattern (fitful sleep, not sleeping or sleeping too much);

3) Loss of interest in activities formerly enjoyed (hobbies, friends, personal appearance, sex);

4) Loss of energy (tired after sleeping, fatigue, too exhausted for routine tasks);

5) Feelings of worthlessness (the world would be better off without you);

6) Feelings of inappropriate guilt (breathing is using air someone else could use, everything

you do seems wrong);

7) Inability to concentrate (thinking muddled, indecisive, read a page and can't remember what it said at the beginning—when you reach the end, you don't care);

8) Recurring thoughts of death or suicide, wishing to die, suicide attempt (planning funeral, writing apology to family or friends for suicide, giving away the good stuff you won't be needing);

9) Overwhelming feelings of sadness (slowed motor skills, grief for what you could have been and loss of control over your life); and,

10) Disturbed thinking (out of touch with facts or reality).

If even three of these symptoms show up on the doorstep of your thinking, it's probably time to take out the trash. Medication may be in order, but there are other ways that have been found helpful in curbing depression if it isn't too deeply set.

The three ways I've found the most consistently useful and effective are:

1) Writing

2) Exercising

3) Leaving the house

If you catch the first red flag, then apply one or all of the above suggestions, there is a good chance that the edge of depression will lift and not descend into clinical depression.

Writing almost anything helps, but a more directed writing is, of course, more beneficial. I use trigger questions to get me going:

1) What is the problem?

2) What would it take to fix it?

3) What feels hopeless?

4) Have I ever felt this way before?

5) What happened?

6) What are the facts?

Feelings are not facts; however, they are very real. Feelings can and do change. Facts do not.

Learning to make decisions based on facts, not feelings, results in better decisions—which can often change feelings.

When I speak of feelings, I'm talking about the emotional, surface reactions to situations and circumstances. You can feel overwhelmed by a mountain of tasks requiring attention, when the fact is, taken item by item, the mountain can be tackled easily and is not more than you can accomplish. Changing the impossible to possible is often the results when feelings and facts are separated.

Another use of the word *feelings* is an underlying reality. For example, whenever I get angry (surface feeling), the underlying reality is fear (feeling or gut-knowledge).

When I speak of "getting in touch with your feelings," I'm referring to that gut-knowledge reality. It is easy to identify your anger. Something is clenched, you feel like throwing anything, you scream at the kids and/or other drivers. Anger is the external expression of fear:

1) of being made to look stupid or inadequate,

2) of potential bodily harm, or

3) of not having power and control in your life.

Anger doesn't accomplish anything constructive. There are three ways to handle anger: get it out, stuff it, or disarm it. By looking below the surface to the spiritual self, I see my inner fear and recognize that without drawing on some inner strength—God, Universal Good or Higher Power—I should be afraid. My track record, alone, is terrible. Yet, every time I've placed myself and/or my circumstances in the care of this Power, the situation has not only become tolerable, it has turned out better than anything I could have conjured up.

A bad situation may not change immediately, but who I become as a result of the difficult time prepares me for what comes next. Sometimes the "bad" thing isn't so bad if my experience benefits others.

Writing "Dear God" letters works for me when I can't get a fix on my problem and know only that I am boiling mad. The letters smooth the way and in the waning moments of depression, I see my own expectations were a long way from any possible reality.

Exercising is not only effective, it is bio-chemically sound for you and for the manic-depressive in your life. It doesn't have to be an all-out marathon or even two hours a day. Formal exercise includes everything: walking, jogging, roller-blading, swimming, biking, weight training, etc. When you take part in any of these activities, you know you're exercising.

For me, exercising also includes vacuuming, mopping or serious housecleaning—anything that produces sweat. I'm not sure if sweating or muscle movement creates the change in my mood, but it works. The biggest problem I face when I need to exercise to overcome the onset of depression is that my brain lies to me and says, "You're too tired," or "It won't work this time." If I don't put up a good fight, I'll sink lower into the depression until I truly can't exercise or write or do anything but sit on the floor in the dark and cry.

We all have our own special manifestation of depression. Most of the people I've talked with say they spend days under the covers and have no energy to even move to the couch. Others sit and stare. Sometimes I curl into a fetal position in the middle of the bed, with or without covers.

Whenever you feel down or mildly depressed, bathing, dressing and getting out of the house is a chore. It seems not only difficult. It feels totally unnecessary. Feelings often mask themselves as facts.

When I worked full time for an attorney, wrote mystery novels and taught two nights a week, it was next to impossible to include exercising in my routine. I often lied to myself and claimed all the walking I did at work counted as exercise. It didn't. I never sweated.

Most of my physical energy goes into stretching, swimming and walking. I do try to be consistent. Even so, some days I ignore the warning flags and all I want to do is curl into a fetal position. If I force myself into an early shower or better yet, a bubble bath, then dress, add a full-scale makeup job and leave the house, by the time I reach the car I find myself in a better mood.

Exercise helps me keep a clear eye and a realistic view of my life.

Bob exercises routinely every day. He alternates jogging with weightlifting and has for years. He is very dedicated to this, and I am very grateful. Sometimes when we have unexpected guests, he leaves us all sitting there and goes for his jog. If they don't understand the importance of this, I don't worry about them being offended.

If I do everything I know to do to minimize the depth and duration of my depression, it usually lifts within a few hours. When I can't (or won't) do any of the above and it lasts for more than a week, I call my doctor. I know when I'm in that state of mind, I won't be able to dig my way out alone. This has happened only three times in ten years. Each time my doctor had a solution: increase or change medication. The one I'd been on had quit working. Keeping in close contact with your doctor or psychiatrist is essential.

Developing my inner strengths has been the most important part of maintaining my emotional equilibrium. I have done this using several avenues:

1) Prayer and meditation

2) Volunteer work

3) Networking

I believe each of us prays in a unique fashion, whether praying in the traditional manner of Christians, Jews, Buddhists, or any other religion—or no organized religion at all. Seeking spiritual answers to life's complex problems is common in all cultures. Most religions recommend a regular morning and evening prayer time. I suggest that however you pray, having a scheduled time is important.

This is not to say you should avoid praying at random times as the need arises. Discipline in spiritual matters seems to have advantages beyond the words or thoughts expressed. I have worked very hard, using a number of ways to help me develop such discipline.

I have also talked with others who are seeking a spiritual path. One woman throws a pillow on the floor at bedtime to kneel on the next morning. She said, "If I don't trip over that darned pillow on the way to the bathroom when I wake up, I miss it. I know I'm going to have to pick it up when I make the bed, and as long as I'm bending over, I may as well say good-morning to God while I'm at it."

Others I've talked with have a special place and time scheduled for after their shower, before coffee, after coffee, before they get dressed, after they get dressed. One man has an inconvenient string tied around his toothbrush as a reminder. When and how is not nearly as important as doing it.

One of the helpful hints I received from a fellow traveler includes keeping a pen and paper close by. If my thoughts wander to something, I write it down and continue my prayers. Often it's something I really need to remember, like picking up the dry cleaning or taking out the trash. If either were left undone, the world would not end, but keeping on top of chores keeps our household running smoothly. And who know, maybe it's God's way of reminding me of what I need to do.

I also keep the pen and pad close at hand when I'm meditating. Rarely do I feel urged to write, however.

Any meditation technique is helpful. Before I go into twenty minutes of meditation, though, I usually read something uplifting. Again, *what* I read is not nearly as important as *that* I read something to my benefit.

If you don't have any inspirational literature on hand, any bookstore clerk will guide you to the right shelf. Look through the offerings and see what strikes a chord with you. This is your own personal journey. It's important to chose a book that you believe will speak to you.

One of my fears was of being caught on my knees. I know it must sound silly to some, but even though my husband and I share much in common on our spiritual journey, we have never prayed together. Many couples do, and I applaud them. For us, it didn't work. Yet, we each have our meditation and prayer routine well established—in separate rooms.

My routine has changed as I've changed. If you make spiritual progress, yours will change, too. Of course, first you have to establish your routine. Five minutes may be all you think you can spend. Or maybe you intend to start a prayer and meditation routine as soon as you find the time. We all have the same number of hours in a day. Even sixty seconds is a good beginning. If you have a timer, set it for one minute. Pray as leisurely as you desire. You'll be surprised how much territory you can cover in only one minute.

Self-esteem is a tricky thing. Like happiness, it's not something I've ever been able to go after and succeed. It is always a by-product of something else, usually doing something I don't want to do but do anyway just because it's right. That's how I got into volunteer work.

Living with a manic-depressive has advantages. I have attended Depressive Manic-Depressive Association (DMDA) meetings with Bob and met other family members who suffer from some of the same frustrations and fears I've experienced. Trying to help them gets me in "service mode," a crucial step toward serenity. It seems as if God fixes me whenever I'm busy trying to help one of His kids.

Anytime I can focus on helping someone else, whether it is formal volunteer work or individually targeted people who appear to need my help, I am not focused on myself and my problems. This gets me out of God's way. And always, when I least expect it, and answer via a phone call, an intuitive thought, a chance meeting gives me the answer, which completely eluded me when I concentrated on the problem.

The other day I couldn't see how I was going to be in three places at once. I'd over committed and knew I had to cancel two appointments. They all seemed equally important. I decided not to decide prematurely. I waited until the day before the scheduled events. Early that morning, I placed the problem in God's hands by writing a "Dear God" letter detailing my thoughts on speaking to a writers group, visiting a friend's son in the hospital and going to dinner with a friend who would only be in town one night.

By ten o'clock that morning, I learned that the young man was going home at noon and his mother thought it best he stay quiet and not have company. My out-of-town friend was unable to conclude her business and called to ask if we could postpone our dinner until the following evening. Problem solved. I gave the talk to the writers, knowing I hadn't neglected something or someone to do it.

I am in no way suggesting God rearranged the lives of other people to accommodate me. If I'd made a decision earlier, I would have been working with less than all the facts. From my perspective, I wanted to dine with my friend and felt obligated to speak to the writers. I also wanted to, and felt strongly that I should, visit the young man in the hospital.

There are also times when I am forced to make a decision between two or more equal endeavors. On those occasions I used to figure if I didn't want to do a thing, it was probably what I should do. I had no concept of God directing my decisions. I, for some obscure reason, thought if I *wanted* to do it, it must be against God's will. After all, isn't everything tasty, fun and fattening immoral or illegal?

God often gives me a desire to do what He wants me to do. A strange concept at first glance. If I ask for guidance, make a decision, then take the action, I have to trust I did what God hoped I'd do. It has been my experience that even if it appears I've screwed up, because my desire to do God's will is so strong, He makes it come out right anyway.

Sometimes it doesn't look or feel right at first. It may take a long time before I understand that the very thing I suspected of being a tragedy was the catalyst for the next obviously wonderful event.

More often than I like to admit, my plans are based on insufficient evidence and my living comes off like a cake baked without any baking power or soda: a real flop. That's my evaluation on a bad day. You know what a bad day is, don't you? It's one that didn't go my way.

Living with a manic-depressive brings on a lot of bad days. Of course, it isn't really the days that are bad. It's my thinking and my evaluation of our situation.

I once called a friend and complained, "Everything that can go wrong has gone wrong today?"

She said, "I'm so sorry you have inoperable cancer and God has left you to cope with it alone."

I replied, "I do not have cancer." I couldn't imagine how she'd arrived at that conclusion.

She purred, "Then everything that could go wrong didn't."

I conceded, counted my blessings and asked how she was holding up. Sometimes lending an ear is volunteer work. If I'd rather be talking about me and I listen to someone else, that's time I'm investing in someone else—voluntarily.

If you look around you at neighbors, church or synagogue friends, strangers in the supermarket, and tune in to what you might be able to do to help, you'll be surprised. I once spent a summer taking a neighbor boy to weekly music lessons. His mother had confided how badly he wanted to go, but she couldn't get off work to take him. Picking him up after the lesson was no problem. I could tell she wasn't hinting. She was really rambling about all the activities her boys craved. We were standing in line at the grocery store.

When I made the commitment, it sounded simple enough. As the weeks wore on, I wondered about my sanity. Many times I did not want to stop what I was doing to take Sam to his music lesson. During that summer I learned something vital: If I want to do it, it is not a sacrifice. When I sacrifice some of my time to help others, my self-respect soars. If I do it because I want to, it's easy, or it makes me look good, I tend to become pious and condescending. Then I'm really in trouble.

One of my core thoughts on volunteer work is that I'm volunteering my time and energy to God, by way of whomever I'm helping.

Organized volunteer programs are wonderful. I particularly wanted to help in a literacy program. However, because of the same reason I can no longer work in a law office, I can no longer commit to any schedule. I never know when I'll have a lupus flare-up and be unable to perform.

If you're inclined toward a particular cause, by all means investigate their needs and see if you can fill any of them. While you're helping others with their problems it is impossible to concentrate on your own. And after all, anything that gets us out of God's way enables Him to work on and in our life. Also, keep in mind that God isn't hard of hearing. Once we ask for help, He knows what we said. If it's in our best interest and not to the detriment of anyone else, it will probably come to pass. Staying out of His way by trying to be of service to others increases the possibility.

Staying out of God's way accomplishes two things: spiritual growth and it puts us in contact with people—which always seems to alleviate our depression if we haven't allowed it to drag us to the very bottom. Then there is a bonus. While we're helping someone else, we're actually living our life. We're no longer focusing on the manic-depressive we love.

There are times, however, when we must focus on the manic-depressive.

# Chapter 4

*When manic, the family wants help and the patient won't get it;*
*when depressed, the patient wants help but can't ask for it —*
                                          *Anonymous DMDA Member*

As we drove away from the little town in the beautiful Texas Hill Country, I asked Bob one simple, direct question. Do we have that much money in the bank?

He had given a realtor a check for $20,000, buying us two more condos in the heart of Texas. The first two were still going in the hole every month. Negative cash flow was a big tax advantage, he explained. And back then, several years before he was diagnosed with bipolar disorder, it was true in some cases.

In answer to my question, he said, "No, but don't sweat it. I'll cover the check in the morning."

And he did!

So why shouldn't I believe him? Why shouldn't I trust him?

It was nothing I could put my finger on, but something didn't make sense to me. I had a Series 7 stockbroker's license, a Group I life insurance license and a realtor's license. I'd also earned three-fifths of a Chartered Financial Counselor designation. I had gathered and stockpiled licenses for ammunition. If I had proof I knew about such things, I'd have logical, intelligent arguments against his rash spending, which he would surely listen to. I knew sinking such a large percentage of our income into real estate was not a smart investment move.

In the realtor's office I had tried to dissuade him from the purchase, but was brushed aside by both men as if I just didn't understand the fine details of high finance. Yes, we were leveraged. It was the only way to go.

While he was still in that manic phase, nothing seemed impossible. Yet, as happy as he sounded, my heart filled with fear and resentment. I wanted to find out what was wrong with him. A question I often posed to myself was, "Where is my Bob?" I knew the man I married lived inside this raving, raging maniacal apparition who stayed up half the night, plotting his rise to fame. He also talked faster, drove faster, made love to me daily, ate faster than our dog and jiggled his knee (or some other part of his anatomy) constantly.

Couldn't anyone else see what I saw? Evidently not. No matter who I tried to discuss my situation with, no one seemed to think I should try to slow down the genius. Maybe he was right after all. Maybe I was crazy. I felt as if the ground shifted with each step I took. He was captivating and frightening. If I was right, and he did need help, I had no idea where look for that help. I had no idea what kind of help he needed. It never occurred to me that I needed help, too.

The higher he went, the more afraid I became. I knew what went up would eventually come down. I didn't know that while he was going up, he was watching himself make foolish decisions and rash statements. All that time he was also wondering why.

During that last big manic episode, I couldn't mention that I liked something or he brought home a case of it. I didn't think I'd ever drink all the cranberry juice he stockpiled because I'd said I liked it. I reached the point where I couldn't stand the thought of another box of Total cereal.

It was the same way with clothing and jewelry. If I saw a blouse I liked, he bought it. If I commented on a diamond ring, he bought it. It never mattered whether we could afford it or whether it was a good buy or whether I really liked it enough to want to own it. Many bipolars are selfish with their money even while they are throwing it away. Bob was not.

My wish was his command. His wish was his command!

He once walked into a store (this was in the 80's) and picked up three shirts he liked. He plunked them on the counter and said, "I'll take these."

When the bill came to over $500, he slapped down a platinum credit card as if he had good sense. After all, he reasoned, I'd recently set him back $700 for a formal evening dress. Besides, there was plenty more where that come from. Five hundred dollars was pocket change.

And that is my point. Everything he did, he had a reason that made sense to him. And I, caught up in the grandeur and fun of it all, bought my share of expensive trinkets. Sometimes I bought to get even. Sometimes I bought to get my share. More importantly, I held my tongue or went so far as to encourage his lavishness, lest I put a hex on him and stop his enthusiasm and fun.

Silently, I wanted the whirling world to stop so I could get off. I wanted him to understand that I loved him, not his money. We'd been married a good many years when all this took place, most of it on a shoestring. I had never wanted to leave him because we were broke, and I never stayed because of the money he made during the eighties.

I knew something was wrong. I knew his behavior was not normal. I didn't know the signs of manic-depression and am not sure I could have done anything about it if I had. I did know I felt afraid.

My fear was more justified than I realized at the time. He was borrowing as much money as he earned. Some of his business transactions were somewhat less than legal. Now I know that this is a common occurrence among bipolars, who are often convinced they are invincible and cannot be convicted or even touched by the law.

The longer he stayed manic, the closer I came to cracking up. Toward the end, I wanted help for me and for him.

It was not long after the condo purchases when he began the slide into the depression that landed him in the hospital. He went from soaring with eagles to looking for a crawfish hole to climb into.

When it became obvious the money had run out, there were days when my resentment knew no bounds. It wasn't that I wanted the sums he'd been bringing in. I wanted to be able make the house payment, the utilities, the basics. I didn't want to go through another eviction; I didn't want to go through bankruptcy. Although I'd done nothing to save any of the money we made, I was angry with him for not providing a livable income. As he got sicker, I got angrier.

I couldn't keep quiet. I seemed to be looking for a fight. One afternoon as he lay on the couch, looking awful and coughing with every other breath, he asked, "Why do you get mad when I'm sick?"

I said, "I'm not mad, just frustrated." In part, that was the truth.

His depression manifested first in respiratory ill-nesses. It was one way his work-ethic background allowed him to stay in bed. Later, there were unre-lenting headaches. He woke up with them and went to bed with them. He seemed to stay sick. I seemed to stay mad.

Although I've experienced clinical depression in recent years, at that time no amount of understand-ing could prepare me for his episodes. Feeling help-less kept me wrapped in anger. The only other time I have felt so completely helpless was when one of my daughters was in the hospital. The doctor was considering a blood transfusion if she didn't keep down at least a small amount of food in the follow-ing twenty-four hours. As afraid and helpless as I felt then, I knew something right was being done for her.

With Bob, I didn't know what to do for him, and at the time, neither did his doctor.

Watching him sit and stare, tears rolling down his cheeks, I wondered if our life would ever be nor-mal. I should not have wasted my time wondering. I should have, instead, used whatever trickery needed to get him to a hospital.

Eventually, that's what I did. A friend calmed me down and took me to Bob's doctor to explain what I was facing. We concocted a plan. The doctor would call the house and tell Bob he had come up with one more test he could do in an attempt to locate his problem. Bob would have to check into the hospital for the test.

It worked. The following day Bob entered the hospital.

And I was very angry. I stayed angry for a very long time.

Since then, I've learned to deal with my anger in several ways. Primarily, I follow the suggestions in the foregoing chapter. Additionally, I have learned several truths, some hard to swallow. The biggest chunk of all is that there may come a time when there is *nothing* I can do to prevent his suicide. It's the nature of the beast.

Most times there is *something* I can do to help him past the slick spots that can send him into that terminal slide toward suicide. Having him hospitalized is a last resort, but I know it is always a consideration, over his objections or not, should nothing else elevate his mood.

At this point, I must interject that Bob has been a willing participant in the maintenance of his own mental health. If bipolar disorder gets the better of him, he counts on me to intervene.

One morning he refused to get up. Knowing he often helped other manic-depressives through rough times, I stood over him and asked, "Is this the same man who tells others to get out of bed unless they're running a fever? Is this the same man who says he *always* runs or works out to keep his sanity?"

I had several more sarcastic questions lined up, but after those two, he threw back the covers. I scrambled out the front door. When I got to the office, I called a mutual friend and asked her to phone him and get back to me.

When I spoke to her again, she said he was grateful I'd been so harsh. He wasn't feeling wonderful, but he'd get to his support group and see if he didn't begin to feel better. He also jogged that evening.

Confronting him is against my nature. It was a result of courage I drew from God, and my belief that Bob truly wanted to maintain his mental health to the best of his ability. Forcing him to get out of bed gave him that opportunity.

That's my job. His job is to take his medication, stay in touch with his doctor, get his blood levels of lithium monitored and follow a plan that includes medication, meditation, exercise and involvement in a support group.

Sometimes I still get angry. My self-centeredness leads me to thinking he could skip exercise "just this once," when we have unexpected company, I want to go to an early movie, I want... I want.... I can even warp the situation around to, "If he loved me, he'd...." That's when I have to take another look at my motives. I can think that I, after all, only want us to be happy, when I know we can never be happy if he doesn't do what he's supposed to do. If I am not supporting him, I'm not supporting us.

If I take care of my attitude, his seems to be much better. Why is that?

Part of taking care of my attitude is to have outside interests. By *outside* I mean other than what we do together. I am interested in foreign languages, and have taken a few classes in Spanish. I like taking classes in almost anything. He likes to be outdoors. I can't take the heat or cold. He likes boating. I like baking. He likes eating. We work well together.

Another part of taking care of my attitude is keeping my mouth shut when he does anything in any way other than the way I would have done it. I have a terrible time with that. I'll probably be working on it with my last breath. If he has generously offered to vacuum, I try to tell him which plug to use. If he's making sandwiches for our lunch, I can hardly keep from telling him how I do it. And I don't intend to go into his driving and my coaching.

When Bob became a "mental patient" I decided he had suddenly become stupid and I had to mother him strongly since he needed my guidance. He claims the mother gene kicked in when our first child was born and I wouldn't get rid of it when they left home. Who knows who's right? It doesn't matter.

He may be crazy, but he's not stupid.

I can't coach from the sidelines and expect him to play his game.

As long as he's committed to being as stable as he can be, there is nothing I won't do to try to monitor my tongue. I've counted to ten. I've silently walked away—mad and otherwise. I've groused to a trusted friend. I've consulted a spiritual advisor. And I've talked when I shouldn't have—always to my regret. I know I'm making progress, though. The last time I wanted to tell him what I thought, I gave him a hug and said, "You'll figure it out."

As long as I keep my own counsel, I do just fine. If you can use a boost in the self-esteem department, try not saying what you think. Try acting your way into the right way of thinking. Act as if you trust that the manic-depressive in your life has some basic common sense from time to time. Every thought and every idea is not necessarily insane. There are some very smart manic-depressives (Lincoln, Churchill, to name a couple). So, listen. It may even be true that there's more to your bipolar than you remember. You evidently saw something in that person or you wouldn't be involved in the first place.

Bipolar disorder does not diminish intelligence. It does produce ruptured relationships within the family. If you have children, there are some things you should know.

# Chapter 5

*What About the Children?*

—*Every mother.*

When it comes to children, the first consideration is their physical welfare. If they are in any danger of being physically abused, get them out of situation immediately. I knew, without any reservations, that Bob would never physically harm ours. He also would never physically abused me.

This is not always the case with bipolars. Many are inclined toward violence. In those cases, I know of no other solution than to leave. If you leave, and the manic-depressive succumbs to the urge to commit suicide, it is not your fault. You are not guilty. It is a terrible illness, but not the only one that kills. Children's safety must come first. Even the manic-depressive in lucid moments will agree.

If you feel guilty for taking the children away from their abusive parent, remember that it is nothing you did to cause the abuse—no matter what the manic-depressive says. You are guilty only *if you stay!*

Beyond that, raising a child with one manic-depressive parent still has a few unique problems.

Once you know your manic-depressive is not going into a rage and harm you or your children, it is best to stay out of the relationship between the children and their manic-depressive parent. You don't have to explain lectures, actions or reactions.

On their own, from a very young age, (before Bob was diagnosed) our children understood that he might change his mind, yell at them for something they hadn't done, or not listen to their explanation of why they did something. They learned to deal with him.

They figured out when to stay out of his way and when to play him like fiddle to get what they wanted. Each child developed his or her own relationship with each of us.

It is still my basic nature to explain their father's actions or moods. The girls remind me to butt out. Our son nonchalantly says, "Oh, Mom, I know how Dad is."

Children adapt very quickly. We sometimes lag behind, trying to force the bipolar to do life the right[1] way.

While we were raising our three children, Bob played with, teased and taught our daughters and son with great zeal. He encouraged them, chastised

---

1 Our right way is not necessarily the manic-depressive's right way.

them, and told them he loved them. He did every-thing other fathers do, only more so. All his emo-tions were exaggerated, including his love, patience and anger.

He got madder than a two-year-old when an object or mechanical device didn't perform up to his demands. We've watched him throw a belligerent hammer that dared to hit his thumb instead of a nail. We've heard him curse a car or lawnmower for refusing to start. We've seen him slam telephone receivers until the phone became useless.

We've also seen him visit a burn victim he hardly knew because he learned the man had few friends and no family. We've watched him patiently comfort a confused and despondent child on his YMCA base-ball team. And many, many times he has talked with other bipolars going through a depressive epi-sode. They know he understands. For him, they get out of bed and meet him for coffee. They trust him. They are all still alive.

His laughter comes easily and heartily. He is uninhibitedly fun. Once we strolled through a mall, pointing at clothes or other items we admired. I made a comment on a red dress, (It's a family joke about how many red dresses and blouses I own). When he didn't respond, I looked behind me. There he was, hunched up at the shoulders, arms swing-ing loosely, hobbling toward me like a gorilla, going, "Huh, huh, huh," with his jaw slung forward. All he needed was a banana.

Being a native son of Texas, he usually wears cowboy boots. Sometimes he walks on his heels with his hands in his pockets, like a kid practicing on stilts. He's also been known to drag a stick or his finger along a wall, toss the dry cleaner's shirt tag on top of the wardrobe, or point his finger and "fire" at geese, ducks or doves (and he's not a bird hunter).

Fortunately, through the years, I've come to believe that his actions do not reflect on me, though sometimes I wish they would. I have a tendency to worry about what people think, or if my actions are the adult way to behave. His childlike (not childish) sense of fun and adventure are delightful.

His ability to make any mundane or normal event into a celebration of fun and life still captivates me. I never know what to expect. As for the reactions of other people, most of them seem to enjoy his antics.

All three of our children have his enthusiasm for life. They have become outstanding adults, readily have spontaneous fun experiences, and demonstrate a result of successful parenting. The truth is, however, God doesn't have any grandchildren. Allowing them to develop their own relationship with a Higher Power gave them a solid grounding.

Of course, they were exposed to regular Sunday school and church from an early age. When they rebelled, we didn't take issue with them. Instead, we trusted that the seeds of faith had been planted deeply. As they grow, their relationship with God has changed, as has mine. They are still searching, growing and changing. As God's kids, I know they will continue to develop a relationship with Him.

So why am I still guilty of trying to change Bob? Because I want to help. I mentioned this earlier, but I have to broach the subject again. It is so subtle and causes so much unnecessary animosity. Recently, he offered to vacuum for me. It is one of those chores that is very difficult for me, especially when lupus flares up in my large muscles or joints.

Wasn't it his sensitivity to my condition that caused him to offer? So why did I point out, as if I were talking to a child, that the cord reaches all three bedrooms if he'd only use the plug in the hallway like I do? Did I really care which plugs he used? Did it make any difference?

Where was my sensitivity? My sense of appreciation?

It is times like this when I must quit blaming him and look at me. If I feel guilty for treating him so rudely, it is because I am guilty! I apologized, of course. Almost immediately. I promised God and myself that I wouldn't try to tell him how to do anything again. And of course, I did. I am guilty of being human. I don't apologize for that. If I'm not making mistakes, I'm not alive. I have asked God to seal my lips and remind me I am not Bob's mother.

I try to refrain from beating myself for goof-ups. If we don't accept our own fallibility, we're not likely to accept anyone else's. Everything manic-depressives do is not because of bipolar disorder. Much of who they are and what they do is a result of their personality, disposition and upbringing. Cut them some slack, especially when it is obvious most of the time that they are doing the very best they can with what they've got, exactly as we are.

So often I want to blame Bob for my state of mind. If I'm uninspired, out of sorts, or tired of doing the same old thing, is it really his fault? Making new friends, visiting new places is up to me. When I want to take the children to a museum, a play, an opera, my first argument is either we can't afford it, or he won't like it. If he won't like it, does that really prevent me from going? I think not. It is merely a good excuse for me to complain.

If we truly can't afford an entertaining excursion, there are many freebies, including nature walks.

Nature walks may include a tour of your own neighborhood, pointing out to the children the variety of plants and trees. Once we went around the block marveling at the differences and similarities of the houses. If your children are culturally deprived, you are as much to blame as the manic-depressive. Do something about it.

When Bob's income dips from time to time, which is not uncommon among manic-depressives, I want to yell or complain about not having what I want *right now*. So what do I do instead? I increase my earnings. When that's not possible, I count my blessings.

I write out a list of things I'm grateful for. Some days it is all I can do to count my fingers and toes. Most days I list the people who are important to me, who have played a part in my life and made it richer.

Next, I list the people I've tried to help. My goal is for the lists to be the same length. I'll never be able to help as many men and women as have helped me, but I'm still trying.

One more word about the children. Research supports that close relatives of manic-depressives are genetically vulnerable for manic-depression.[2] Because the potential is there, please do not assume all your children will have bipolar disorder.

Yes, take note of their moods. But children's moods normally swing erratically. Don't label them manic-depressive prematurely. It may never happen. It is a good idea to enlist their cooperation in coping with their moods. Ask questions.

Could you have handled that differently?

What do you think the problem is?

I know you're angry. What can you do to feel better?

I know you feel tired. What do you think would give you energy?

---

2  According to Charles Nemeroff of Emory University in Atlanta, Georgia.

It is possible that your child will be diagnosed in his or her late teens. Dropping
out of school is not uncommon at the high
school or undergraduate level. Making big
plans that cannot be followed is also stan-
dard procedure. Then there are the temper tantrums, withdrawal into their own
room and refusing to take part in family
outings.

These activities can also be an indication of drug
or alcohol problems, thyroid problems, teen rebel-
lion or complete normalcy.

If you suspect bipolar illness or chemical
dependency, get medical attention for your child any
way possible. If a medical condition is diagnosed,
make sure your child follows doctor's orders. As a
parent, you're completely within your rights to
demand watching him or her take the prescribed
medication. You not only have the right, you have the
responsibility. It would, of course, be better for both of
you if the bipolar were eagerly medication compliant.

There may come a time when your child threat-
ens to run away or exhibits other self-destructive
behavior. You can only do what you can do. No more.

Even if the genes carrying the manic-depressive
tendency came from you, it is not your fault. You
cannot force your teenaged child to take medication
or instill values he or she refuses to accept. The
more you push, the angrier and more strongly the
child will rebel.

Remember that much of what you say and do is still seeping in. The groundwork is laid. As children mature, what they understand, what they are willing to do for their own health changes. You don't know what your child must go through to get where he or she is going.

With younger children it may be necessary to try distracting them when they are angry. You can also encourage a balance of physical activity and rest. Anything you can do to help a child feel he or she has control over their life and their moods is a step in the right direction.

Another important step you can take is to listen. Don't try to solve every problem a child brings up. Don't judge their information. Just listen.

I probably know more about skateboarding and photography than most moms. I also know all the super heroes and their powers. The only questions I asked during our afternoon discussions were, "Then what happened?" and "How do you do that?"

One of our children has been diagnosed with depression and minor (or hypomanic) cycles, but not a clear case of bipolar disorder, but at this time is not on medication with doctor approval. One is very stable, focused and dependable. One may have trouble in later years, but has developed a system to control the mood swings to within safe limits. All three are opinionated, outgoing, and have a strength born of perseverance, a trait they got from their father.

Since I do not know what my children have to go through to get where they're going, my advice now that they are out of the nest and on their own is not only wasted, it is not appreciated. Giving advice is also one more way to say I don't think I did a good job. One more way to try to change someone other than myself.

I bite my tongue when one of my offspring seems to be on the wrong track, and I somehow mysteriously *know* (mind-reading?) how to redirect him or her. Am I trying to force them onto my track? Or the track I wish I'd taken? Self-analysis at this point is self-defeating. Your motive need not be an issue. Simply stop. Stop trying to help when your help is not requested.

Take my word for it, others, including your adolescent or grown children, have all the tools they need to build their own life. If they're not making mistakes, they're not doing anything. If they're not doing anything, you are not responsible for that, either.

# Chapter 6

*Responsibility: The ability to respond appropriately.*
*—An Alanon Member*

*I* have never been guilty of not responding to Bob or anyone else. How I respond is my problem. An inappropriate response can be worse than no response, and some days that's the best I can do.

I'm using the words *respond* and *react* interchangeably because my response was always my reaction.

My first *reaction* is my *response*. Whether I'm responding to a question or my opinion of someone's actions, the appropriateness is critical to my being understood and to my understanding. When I respond in an inappropriate manner, I am usually guilty of judging whether or not the other person is capable in some area.

Out of fear of bringing on an episode, many spouses and loved ones decide constant vigilance regarding the bipolar is required. Sincerely wanting only what is best for the person, coupled with an over-inflated opinion of self-importance, we nag, quiz and/or demand that they keep us apprised of their comings and goings, thoughts and moods. We think if we know, we can prevent disaster. Whenever we don't know, we foolishly believe we have lost control.

The truth is we never had control—not over our life, not over the manic-depressive's.

Here's a news bulletin I was fortunate to comprehend: If you can't cause it, you can't fix it.

If you think you are in full control of yourself and your life, look back over the past few days. Did everything go the way you planned or expected? Did anything? We don't want something to happen that will drive the patient into the mental and emotional condition that caused the previous hospitalization. Yet, we can't prevent it.

Additionally, we're not responsible for anyone else's mental and emotional health. We can help by being supportive, not nosey, but each person is responsible for his or her own life. Since each life is comprised of thoughts and actions over which we have limited or no control, it behooves us to look to our own lives. Where can we do better? Is our thinking muddled? Do our thoughts center on how to change the bipolar in our lives or how to help? Do we keep our actions thoughtful, patient? Or pushy, manipulative?

Only you know the answers.

There is one arena where we have complete control. That is our ability to develop spiritually. There, we have all the power in the universe. There, we can develop a relationship with God that will become the Power we draw upon, regardless of what is going on around us. Still, we are human.

We all have our auto-pilot control phrases. One such reaction is telling a child, "Be careful, don't spill the juice." That child fully intends to be as careful as possible. He or she doesn't want to spill it any more than you want it spilled. The words are totally unnecessary. How much better it would be to say, "If you look at the glass after each step, you will be able to carry it to the table without spilling it." *Be careful* gives a child the impression that you don't believe he can get it to the table without a spill. It says you believe the child won't be as careful as possible without your coaching.

Telling a manic-depressive, "You better take a jacket. It's chilly out," says you believe the bipolar patient is too "crazy" to know when to dress warmly. An adult, manic-depressive or not, does not need your input (or mine) on the basics unless there is brain damage from some other source.

They also do not need to be reminded to take their medication. Or do they? Since they, too, are human, they are capable of forgetting.

Our fear that our bipolar will have to go back into the hospital can be great. The chances are that your manic-depressive will return to the hospital, possibly as often as twice a year. It may be because he or she quits taking the prescribed medication.[3]

This is upsetting to you, understandably. Can you do anything to prevent it? I don't know. Each case is different.

I have used several methods to prevent Bob from feeling like a wayward child and still find out if he's taken his meds. I suspect he knows when I do it. I say, "Gosh, I think I forgot to take my vitamins." This, of course, reminds him if he forgot to take his lithium. It takes a load off my mind; it saves face for him.

At other times, usually when our routine is changed by eating out or being on a trip, I will bluntly ask, "Did you take your medicine?" I do, however, have reminding rights.

About a year after Bob had been on medication he forgot, completely forgot to take his pills for two evening doses in a row. I didn't realize what had happened, but I asked him on the third night if he'd taken his meds. He said, "I'm not a kid, you know. I can take care of my own medications." Then he opened the cabinet, and with one glance, he realized there were more pills in the bottle than there should have been.

We had a discussion, mostly calm, and I asked, "Would you give me permission to ask if you've taken your medicine? Maybe it would keep this from happening again, and I don't want to be a nag."

---

3 Taking medication as prescribed does not guarantee no return to the hospital. See Chapter 11.

He agreed. Reminding rights granted, I don't feel like a nag and he doesn't feel like an incompetent child.

I do not believe I can sit idly by, knowing he has merely forgotten, not deliberately quit taking his meds. My fears of his potential crisis forces me to make decisions that are completely unnecessary for other wives, even wives of alcoholics or addicts. I cannot detach, with or without love. I must be aware without hovering, involved in the maintenance of his mental health without assuming responsibility for it.

A tightrope? Definitely. But not impossible.

I quickly learned that other people also held my fear of doing something wrong. A week or so after Bob got out of the hospital, one of my aunts was in town visiting my mother. Mother called to be sure it would be advisable for them to come by for a quick visit. In her words, "We don't want to undo anything."

Their fear of "undoing" something was real and very strong. Neither of the two women had ever been around anyone who had been in a psychiatric hospital. They care about Bob and were, in their opinion, wanting only to do what was best for him. They had no concept of how little power they had over him and his recovery.

Bob later said he'd had to control a terrible urge to throw himself on the floor, convulsing and slobbering in front of them. We giggled for days over what their reaction would have been. A warped sense of humor? Maybe. We have found that a sense of humor sees us through many tough times.

In this role of not assuming responsibility for the actions of the manic-depressive, one of the problems you may encounter is sexual dysfunction. When this happens, it is usually for one of two reasons: medication or depression.

It is very important for your future sex life that you *do not* assume responsibility for the dysfunction, nor should you place blame in his or her lap, so to speak. I would advise you to remind your partner that medication could be the problem. Do not mention that you feel like a failure, an unsexy partner who cannot turn-on anyone. You may feel that way, but that is most likely not a fact.

Encourage your mate to discuss this problem with the doctor. There are several anti-depressants, often used in conjunction with lithium or other medications, which have the side effect of decreasing libido and/or inhibiting ejaculation.

Lack of interest in sex is often a symptom of depression, which also needs to be addressed by the doctor. Many anti-depressants are on the market today. It may take some trial-and-error investigation, but the doctor will work with the bipolar patient until an acceptable medication is found.

Sometimes it can be as simple as changing the time of day the medication is taken.

I once called Bob's doctor, explained our problem and said, "This won't do. What are our options?"

He laughed and said, "Have Bob call me and we'll find another anti-depressant."

When I relayed the message, Bob did as instructed. Then several weeks later, when life seemed to be back to satisfactory, he got furious that I'd called his doctor with such a delicate problem.

I apologized, but the damage had been done. I'd assumed responsibility—his responsibility—and I was wrong. What I'd done was essentially to say I didn't believe our sex life was important to him.

A few years later, when another anti-depressant quit working and depression interfered with his sexual performance, I gently (or so it seemed to me) said, "Maybe there's something the doctor can change to make a difference. Maybe you should give him a call."

He glared at me. "That's what I plan to do. If you'd just trust me a little, it would help."

He was right, again. I hadn't given him time to act responsibly. I'd had to hover, coach and s/mother. That's smother, my misplaced mothering and a sign I'm not thinking of him as a competent adult. As I said earlier, crazy doesn't mean stupid.

Of course, intellect has no bearing on manic-depression. The slow of mind as well as the brilliant

can inherit the gene that makes someone suscepti-
ble to bipolar disorder.

One of the symptoms I've noticed in many
manic-depressives is that they think too much.
They will worry over a simple comment for days or
even years. They can take a phrase and twist it,
review it, re-live the conversation, and twist it
again. Grudges seem to linger and forgiveness
seems a foreign concept. Those who are willing to
forgive, who actually forgive and who try to grow
spiritually still have problems with relationships at
all levels.

Since bipolars can also have a paranoid flavor,
many will often take the attitude of "do unto others
before they do unto you." While aggressive behavior
is not limited to bipolars, they see it as their defense
against possible or imagined attacks. Being with a
bipolar in such a state may cause very awkward
social situations.

Do not take responsibility for the manic-depressive's social adaptation.

If you try, it will make you crazier and more frustrated than you can imagine, unless, of course,
you've already tried that tack. In that case, you
know exactly what I'm referring to. The situation,
as you see it, is seen in a totally different light by
the manic-depressive. Yet the bipolar is certain he
or she is right. You will never convince the person
otherwise. Don't even try. It will only cause an argument if you do.

The hardest part of following the above instructions is not explaining anything to anyone, not the other people involved, and certainly not the manic-depressive in your life. This is not a matter of who's right and who's wrong. It is a matter of perception. You can't explain away someone else's perception of a situation.

Most of the bipolars I know, men and women, have a somewhat pugilistic nature. I heard one young woman say, "I think a day is wasted if I haven't been in a fight with at least one person."

She got a manic and/or adrenaline boost when she fought with co-workers. The rush was worth getting fired repeatedly. Proving she was right by aggressive behavior was more important to her than believing she was right.

Another area of responsibility I have a tendency to take on is picking up and straightening up after Bob. I don't think any of this is related to him being bipolar. More likely it's a guy thing. What happened, though, is that I saw it as another example of his unstable mental state, and set about to fix it. While doing so, I seriously chastised myself for closing his closet door, replacing toilet tissue on the roller in his bathroom, closing cabinet doors and dresser drawers, carrying his glass or coffee cup from the TV room to the sink and, in general, acting as if he couldn't remember basic household courtesy.

What I discovered after several years of frustration, was that I had known a fact and called it a feeling. The fact is that he doesn't remember, care or deliberately avoid such tasks. They are not important to him. If he, strictly by chance, realizes he's left a cup in the living room, he automatically carries it to the kitchen. He is by nature a thoughtful person.

The fact is that I like those things done immediately whenever possible. I do them now for me, not because he doesn't do them. The shift in my attitude makes a tremendous difference in the local atmosphere.

Before this truth came to me, I slammed his closet door and anything else he'd left open or in disorder. Now I smile and gently take care of it. If possible, when he can't see me do it. I do it with a smile for me and compassion for him. I know in my heart that he would never consciously do anything *at* me except build his dish-towers. The dish-towers have become a symbol of his independence and never fail to give him an impish little grin. It's almost a love note, now.

I've learned to dismantle his handiwork before I turn on the tap.

That is an *appropriate* response.

So often a mentally ill person will curse the ones who have tried to help, blame others for the way he or she feels, and say and do things that seem completely wrong. A cancer patient, someone who has diabetes or another long-term physical illness may react the same way. Would you be understanding and compassionate? Could you see that their distress is a result of their illness?

Since mental illness doesn't readily show, we sometimes forget that bipolar disorder is a physical dysfunction of the brain. The affected person truly has a long-term, potentially fatal, physical illness.

I try to remember this when my fuse is short and my bones are tired. Those are the days when no response may be the most appropriate response.

# Chapter 7

*Go with the flow, but don't get wet*

—*Anonymous Penguins*

All our lives we've been encouraged to plan for the future. Set goals. Work toward our goals. Make plans for the weekend. Plan our day. Plan our evening. Plan our work and work our plan. Many appointment calendars are available today, from simple daily notebooks to elaborate computer programs. They are wonderful for most people.

They don't work for me.

None of them allow for the unpredictable chaos scattered throughout the year as a result of living with someone who has bipolar disorder. I do use a calendar for appointments I hope to keep, but I'm not tied to it.

"Be flexible," most serious planners suggest. They never say how flexible.

There may come a point when flexibility means you have to abandon your hopes, desires, hobbies and any idea of a serene future. You may even do so willingly.

Joe prided himself on being flexible. Milly's bipolar illness wasn't going to get him down. He stayed ready to hitch up the boat, rush her to the hospital, beat his last year's sales record, take her for a stroll or clean up after her. He wanted to be all things to her and keep his business going, too. He knew he couldn't, but he was determined to try.

About three years into their marriage, Milly wanted a divorce. Joe asked, "How could she want out? I do everything I can for her. I love her."

Later, Milly told me, "He treated me like I couldn't do anything, but was in charge of everything. He quit acting like a husband and started acting like a servant."

No matter how flexible Joe tried to be, he never had a chance to finish anything he started because he dropped it as soon as she muttered a desire for anything.

That much flexibility can leave you so undirected you feel like a shadow following the moods of the manic-depressive in your life. Like Joe, you can lose who you are and become a virtual slave to the bipolar's moods. Suppressing the essence of you, the part of you who peers out at the world from your eye sockets, can destroy any chance of you building a solid foundation for your relationship.

Too much flexibility can destroy, but too little is equally damaging. A rigid plan, followed as closely as possible, will still demand a modicum of flexibility. Life happens while we're making other plans.

The question is: How do you go with the floe without getting wet?

This brings us back to the truth that disputes the saying I mentioned earlier. "If you do the same thing and expect different results, you're crazy." That makes sense in a sensible world. In the world of bipolar disorder, "If you do the same thing, you'll never get the same results, and that will make you crazy."

So what choice do you have? You can go with the flow, trying to remember that most of the time when the bipolar is following directions, taking medication, exercising, working or doing volunteer work, life may remain fairly stable. With both of you trying to do it right, there will still be other times when no matter how hard the two of you work, bipolar disorder will ruin plans, hurt feelings, alter goals and redirect your thinking.

Your moods, anyone's moods can do the same. No matter how hard we try, we never grow above human. To expect smooth, orderly days every day, that is insanity.

One of the ways I exercise my flexibility is by driving to the store or school or work by a different route. It seems like a trivial change, but I see different buildings, different people. My thoughts are triggered in different directions. An old building I passed recently reminded me of a warehouse I used to pass on the bus going to junior high. That thought led me to revisit memories of how I felt then: scared, skinny and stupid.

Looking back, I know the only word that did not apply was stupid. I had the nasty habit of judging my insides against other people's outsides. I could see my inadequacies very clearly. Everyone else looked perfect.

Those memories caused me to evaluate my current opinion of myself. At this stage of my life, on the days life isn't feeling friendly, I decide I'm "old and ugly, and fat and dumb." I suspected I had, once again, fallen into my old habit. I knew I didn't measure up to perfection, but I'd assumed everyone else did. Silly me.

Another move I try when I need to be more flexible is to look at my job or daily endeavors. Am I trying to do too much? Do I hate what I'm doing? Am I afraid of getting fired? Am I making new friends? Am I staying in contact with old friends?

If I am really walking on egg shells and quaking every time I see my boss, it's time to recall how I got the job in the first place. I was looking for a job. That's how I got it. This realization forces me to equate looking with getting when it comes to jobs. If I was looking for a job when I got this one, if I lose this one and go looking for another, I'll more than likely get another job. More importantly, I remind myself that the job, any job, is merely a channel for God to deliver my earthly needs. If one channel closes, another will open. The source will never run dry, but continue to flow and find new channels.

When you think you're in a rut, you probably are. It is not the bipolar's fault, no matter what you think, any more than his or her illness is your fault. We get in ruts because they are familiar. Most of us are lazy to the marrow. We'll keep doing life the same way instead of taking the initiative. Getting off our duff takes energy. Spending energy creates more energy, whether it's mental or physical.

Break out of your rut. Make new friends. Where? Take a class in something you have always wanted to learn more about: photography, ceramics, knitting, history, philosophy or yoga. Stretch your mind or stretch your body, but quit blaming your mate for your mental attitude or your physical condition.

Another way I reprogram my thinking is to stand in front of a mirror and introduce me to myself as my best friend. Sounds silly, but I've learned a lot about me doing this exercise. I tell the mirror all my best qualities. Sometimes I have to really reach to come up with any good points. Sometimes I get the giggles, a very mood-lifting experience, when I name certain features and call them good. For instance, I have reasonably square shoulders, high cheekbones, and long legs. I also have a bigger belly than I like, but I claim it as an asset. It did the work of carrying three babies and looks it. Do I love it? You bet. Do I feel silly telling myself my belly is a feature I'd want to tell a new friend about? You bet.

Some mornings I wink at the self in the mirror and say, "Not bad for an old broad." I don't mean this as a put-down at all. I figure aging has benefits I'm only now approaching and the "not bad" is definitely delivered as an understatement.

All of this dramatic silliness helps me stay flexible. Life is too critical to take it too seriously. Inviting a friend to meet me for dessert or coffee on short notice throws me into high gear. I dress and powder my nose quickly, eager for the break in my day. I scoop up a paperback novel, or new pictures of the children, or any trinket. Sometimes I take a hastily written poem or short story. I think of whatever I take as my Show-and-Tell.

After a rearrangement of my plans in such a fashion, I realize that friendships are more important than whatever it was I had planned to do.

Being flexible also means that when you get home all excited about the good things that happened during your day and your bipolar that sounds as if he or she is talking from a deep well of depression, you don't panic. Knowing another person is depressed, even when it's someone you love, does not have to dampen your spirits or drag you down to their emotional state.

It may indicate you need to change the plans for the evening. You could invite someone over, or rent a comedy movie, or just let the bipolar hole up. The latter is not usually a good choice, but whatever you decide, make a decision. Don't let it just happen.

Flexibility can be fun or it can ruin your outlook on life. Go with the flow.

Or change the direction of the flow.

When I dared invite another couple over without telling Bob (he had said he didn't want company) I held my breath. When they arrived he was initially irritated. As time passed, very slowly for the first fifteen minutes, I felt sure I'd made a mistake and played the wrong card. I whipped up a quickie dessert and coffee, encouraged Bob to tell them about a humorous incident he'd been through recently, and pasted on a smile that felt as if it didn't fit.

When the couple left two hours later, Bob had leveled off and appeared to have enjoyed the visit. I hadn't done the chores or called about a new class I was slated to teach, but those things could wait. Our relationship could not.

Now, I ask you, was that manipulation? Of course it was. With premeditation, the cooperation of a woman friend, and flexibility, I helped Bob maintain his mental health. The depression had not reached the depth it could have if I'd done nothing. He knows it. I know it. There is nothing wrong or co-dependent in what I did and continue to do. It is done with love and honesty. I honestly want whatever is in his best interest because, ultimately, it is in our best interest.

There have been times when I've taken that same action and he has stayed in the bedroom, only to sink lower into a depression which eventually required medical attention. If I'd acted sooner would it have made a difference? I don't know. I do know I don't kick myself when that happens. I don't get wet with tears or anything else. I just go with the flow.

As you can see, going with the flow requires action sometimes and no action at others. While I don't want to be responsible for his moods, there are days when that is my job because he can't respond to life in his usual manner.

As a rule, I'm very independent. Going with the flow when you're primarily dependent on someone else changes everything and it changes nothing. It is still necessary to take each task, each emotion as it comes. There is no way to rush out and do or feel a week's worth of either.

I learned a lot about being dependent a few years ago. It used to be hard for me to ask for help. When I had surgery on my left ankle to take care of a ruptured tendon, I spent a few months in a wheel-chair. I am strong willed and like my independence. With Bob pushing me almost everywhere I went, I felt unnecessary, a burden. Trying hard to maintain my independence, I insisted on doing certain things, including wash the dishes. It was awkward and messy from the chair, but I wanted to feel useful and do what I could.

Bob wanted to help. I felt as if he wanted to help too much. I'm sure he feels that way about me from time to time. But when I came to something I simply could not do, I learned to ask for help. The experience made me very aware of going with the flow. I tried to go with the reality of the moment. Sometimes it meant asking a stranger to open an especially heavy door. Sometimes it meant asking a friend to push me into a rest room.

Asking for help is not easy for most of us, but I have a theory. Helping someone is such a lift for me. If I don't ask for help when I need it, I'm denying someone else that great uplifting feeling.

I do know that the experience of being so dependent brought to life my worst nightmare: Me in a wheelchair being pushed by a crazy man. It turned out that it went like a dream. He was so concerned and so helpful.

Maybe we're in tune more than most couples. I don't think so, but if we are, it is because we each try to really listen. Have you ever noticed that our language has two separate words? *Listen* and *hear*. You can hear words, noise, and music without really listening. You cannot listen without hearing, but listen implies a deeper understanding. Listen to the bipolar. He or she can tell you what's going on, how they feel, what they want. Too often we read something into the words that isn't there and isn't intended to be implied.

Sometimes just to be sure my listening has been thorough, I repeat what he says in my own words. I am amazed how wrong I can be.

There are days when what he says makes no sense whatsoever. I may be wrong on what I understand, but even with clarification, I can't figure out what he means. If I ask questions or state an opinion, it is taken as argumentative. I rarely say anything during that sort of conversation. I just go with the flow. My few grunts may pass for agreement. I'm not worried about him thinking I agree with him when I don't. The honest truth is that I place more importance on the fact that I love him. If it develops into an argument, we surrender to the entity of our marriage, not to each other.

I don't have to be disagreeable just because I disagree. It is not important for him to know I don't agree, though sometimes he intuitively does. Here, I'm talking about anything from personal preferences to social issues, politics to religion. I try to stay flexible about when and if I state my opinions.

It took time to reprogram my responses from having to tell Bob and anyone who would listen exactly what I thought about any subject. That is a common occurrence when we are searching and trying to firm up our beliefs and opinions. Once they are truly ours, we don't have to defend, argue or express them. We know. When we know, we can freely allow others to differ and have their own beliefs and opinions.

The goals I set these days are far different than the ones I used to set. I have a few general goals and desires: lose ten pounds, write the next chapter of whichever book I'm working on, write two letters a month to each of our children. These and other simple, attainable goals are not time-sensitive, in spite of the letter-writing goal. They are what I'd *like* to do as my life allows.

If I never lose those last ten pounds, I'll still have enough clothes that fit. If I never write another book, the world will keep spinning. If I don't manage to write the letters, I can pick up the phone and call. I do not get disappointed in myself if I don't reach all my goals, or any of my goals. I like to write them down and have a general idea of where and what is important to me. Still, nothing is as important as today.

One exercise I use to get me back into right now, in the present and in touch with who and where I am is to wash the dishes by hand. As I wash each plate, I feel the soapiness slide over the stoneware. I note the temperature of the water, the texture of the sponge or dishrag, the pressure of the running water as I rinse each dish, the weight of the dish. All this concentration on the now also makes me aware of so many miracles: breathing, muscles holding me up and moving my hands and arms, etc.

I often tune in on the now when I'm on the phone or sitting at my computer. It drags me back to now and shuts out apprehension and wishful thinking about the future. I feel my weight in the seat, the keyboard or telephone receiver, the clothes I'm wearing against my skin. And right now, everything is exactly as it is, no better and no worse than the results of my decisions. I'm doing what I'm doing and I'm all right now, as all right as anyone can be.

And so are you.

# Chapter 8

*To Tell or Not To Tell... That Is The Question*
*—A Bipolar's Wife.*

*T*his book exposes my life and Bob's not only to friends, but to strangers as well. The decision to write it did not come easy. It was not until we found ourselves juggling our time and energy, trying to help other bipolars and bipolar magnets that I decided it was time to get it all down on paper.

Most information available on bipolar disorder addresses problems faced by the bipolar and/or goes into great detail about how family and loved ones can help the person with bipolar disorder. We found nothing for family members and loved ones to help themselves remain stable, secure and somewhat in their right minds.

We spent a great deal of time evaluating what the impact of this book might be on the rest of our family. How much did we really want them to know? In the interest of alleviating the aloneness for people who are helplessly in love with someone who is bipolar, we decided there was nothing we could do but proceed. Most of our family knows all about our adventure into the world of manic-depression. As for friends, they understand or they aren't really friends, are they?

It is strangers we hope to reach, those friends we haven't met yet, and who are hanging on by a thin thread. We hope this book will give them the emotional strength that will help them understand the bipolars in their lives. More than that, however, we hope it will lead them to a better understanding of themselves, their relationship and what they can expect in the future.

Many people who love manic-depressives don't want anyone to know they have a mental patient for a friend or loved one. Those are the ones in hiding. Hopefully, after reading this, they won't feel as if they must hide.

I know a few bipolars who do not want even their families to know of their diagnosis. A young woman named Rose comes to mind. She is terrified that her brother will find out her "nervous breakdowns" are really bipolar disorder. When he comes to town, she is afraid that taking her medication will make her seem too calm and he will suspect. Yet, every time she quits taking it, she has to be returned to the hospital.

Returning to the hospital, sometimes several times a year, is not uncommon for manic-depressives. It is most often caused by the bipolar stopping medication against medical advice. The reasoning goes like this: "I'm feeling really good. I don't think I need this stuff anymore." Or, "I'll show him/her nobody can make me take this medication." Or, "I'm just going to quit taking it for a few weeks so I can go manic and make a lot of money."

Another frequent excuse is lack of money to pay for prescriptions, yet there are county services in most areas that can be utilized. Being afraid people will find out is, unfortunately, also high on the list of reasons.

I know some bipolars who live in fear that a boss, co-worker or friend might find out their awful truth. My heart aches for them. Their attitude keeps them sicker than they have to be. As long as they keep their bipolar disorder a secret, they will continue to believe it is something to be ashamed of, something to hide. It will be increasingly hard for them to accept treatment, maintain a medication regime, and do what is necessary to improve and maintain their mental health.

Mental illness of this type is not a weakness or a result of immoral or amoral behavior. It can certainly perpetrate binges of immorality: stealing, driving over the speed limit, infidelity, excessive spending that can lead to writing insufficient checks, and more, much more. Manic-depressive disease is not brought on by the behavior of the person. The disease brings on the unwanted behavior.

So why the big secret? Would you or your bipolar be ashamed if the subject were diabetes?

What about chickenpox? Any fear there? Chickenpox causes itching, which causes scratching. Scratching does not cause chickenpox. That's not a secret. No one I know of blames anyone for scratching when they itch. These days, doctors prescribe medication, which decreases the desire to scratch. Lithium or other medications are prescribed for bipolar disorder. It changes the desire to act in unacceptable, unhealthy ways.

In truth, we are as sick as our secrets. This holds true, as far as I know, for everyone. Living life as if it were an open book is tremendously freeing. There is no worry about anything getting found out, no fear of being banished to the farthermost corner of the earth. An open life entails responsibilities, which I'll go into later, but the freedom from fear is, by far, the biggest advantage.

Anyone, who is afraid of others finding out what they are doing, probably knows they shouldn't be doing such things. If you followed me through a day or a week, you might be bored or surprised or pleased or impressed or shocked, but I would still be able to look you in the eye at the end of our time together. I don't do anything I have to hide. I don't consider myself a saint for staying with Bob. I don't consider myself insane for staying with him. I am not ashamed to tell anyone I'm married to a mental patient. I wouldn't bat a lash at telling anyone he had chickenpox, either. Would you?

He has told me he feels the same way. If he can't talk about it, he can't overcome it.

In the early days right after he was released from the hospital, I hesitated to tell anyone I'd married a mental case. What would they think of my judgment? What would they think of me? Later, I didn't want to tell anyone about Bob's "problem" so it could be strictly his business. As we've gone through the years, we've gradually learned that no matter what we thought would happen when we exposed our dark secret, we were wrong.

There have been perks we never imagined.

One of the benefits of us being open about his illness is that no matter when or where either of us divulges the information, someone invariably comes up and tells him or me about their experience with bipolar disorder, or their parent's or friend's or in-law's. When the person who approaches is the one who has bipolar disorder, he or she always seems relieved to learn that someone else is trying to live a normal life under their same circumstances.

It is only by being open about the illness in our family that we can be of help to other families. I collect information on what to expect from treatment and what not to expect. I read articles and books as soon as they hit the stands. The librarian at our nearest library sometimes calls me when a new book arrives which contains information on bipolar disorder.

I have learned not to expect treatment to make him perfect. If he ever gets perfect, he surely wouldn't want to live with me or any other human on this planet.

I believe strongly in gathering reliable knowledge about the illness. The more you know, the less easily you can be surprised or frightened by symptoms, blood levels or emotional outbursts. The more you know, the more easily you can adapt and go with the flow. More importantly, the more you know, the more families and friends you can help. The more people you help, the more people will know that this particular mental illness (and probably most) is a chemical deficiency in the brain and not a personality or environmental maladaptation to life because of "poor coping skills" (whatever that means).

Because I live life like an open book, I have the responsibility to share what I've learned about bipolar disorder with others. I search for information through many avenues. In addition to the library, I also visit Internet sites. At the time of this writing, the site with the most current and helpful information is www.pendulum.org. There are many good articles there, and many of the book references in this chapter came from their lists.

I know I can never fully understand all the emotions and strange logic of bipolars, but knowing more about the brain dysfunction helps me to be more compassionate.

The following books have been helpful for understanding the manic-depressives in my life:

*An Unquiet Mind, Memoirs of Moods and Madness*, (Alfred Knopf, 1995). This autobiography of psychiatrist Kay, Ph.D., is about identifying and coping with her own manic depression. It is written in layman's terms and provides excellent information about the disease and insight into the workings of the manic-depressive's mind. I read this one after Bob finished it. He told me it was the only book he'd ever seen on bipolar disorder that explains exactly how he thinks and feels.

*A Brilliant Madness, Living with Manic Depressive Illness*, Patty Duke Aston's biography, written with Gloria Hochman (Bantam, 1992). She talks frankly about her out-of-control mania and its taming with lithium. The book contains helpful information about the disease and its control.

*Depression: What Families Should Know,* Elaine Fantle Shimberg. This medical writer has researched and presented a valuable resource for the "other" victims of depression—the loved ones of the sufferer.

*We Heard the Angels of Madness: One Family's Struggle with Manic Depression*, Diane and Lisa Berger, (Marrow, 1991). Forwarded by Alexander Vuckovic, MD, this is the story of one family and how they found help for their nineteen-year-old son.

*Waking Up, Alive*, by Richard Heckler. His story of depression and attempted suicide.

*Understanding Depression*, by Donald Klein, MD and Paul Wender, MD.
*You Are Not Alone*, by Julia Thorne with Larry Rothstein.

*Genetic Studies in Affective Disorders,* Wiley-Interscience, 1994, contains Demitri F. Papalos's contribution, "The Family Psychoeducational Approach." It details genetic heredity inherent in the illness and family tendencies. I have read only the excerpt by Papalos and found it very interesting, in spite of its medical jargon.

*Questions and Answers about Depression and its Treatment,* by Dr. Ivan Goldberg, (The Charles Press, 1993).

*You Mean I Don't Have To Feel This Way?* By Collette Dowling (Bantam Books, 1993).

These books and articles will add to your store of information. It is important to remember that not all bipolars are equal. The illness comes in varying stages and severity. By reading a wide range of literature on the subject, you will be armed with information that will serve you well in the coming years.

Bipolar disorder is not static. It changes faces, it cycles, and it can go into remission. Your perceptions and responses to the changes will determine the quality of your life. That is why it is so important to get the best education on the subject you can.

There are many more volumes written, but those will get you started. As you can see, more has been written about coping with the depressive cycle of bipolar disorder than the manic cycle of the disease because it is during depression that a bipolar is the most likely to become suicidal. Preventing fatalities is critical. Learn the following do's and don'ts. Trust them. Apply them.

1. Do tell the bipolar you love him or her.

2. Don't expect him or her to acknowledge the statement.

3. Do encourage the depressed person to eat.

4. Don't force the issue.

5. Do maintain as near normal a schedule as possible.

6. Don't threaten, cajole or order the bipolar to "snap out of it."

7. Do tell the person, "We'll get through this together," (if you mean it).

8. Do call the doctor immediately if you even suspect the bipolar is having any thoughts of suicide.

9. Don't sound or act disgusted even if you feel that way.

10. Do use any trick you know to get the bipolar out of the house or to the doctor or committed to a hospital if the depression continues.

11. Don't cut off your friends or use the bipolar's depression as an excuse to avoid life.

12. Do write, pray and maintain your own mental health.

There are, of course, other do's and don'ts you will discover on you own. Apply them, too.

You may feel as if you're all you've got. It may even be true. But manic-depression, like life, has a way of changing. The mountaintop of the next change that brings you much joy could not happen without the valley.

Cross the valley like you live life: One day at a time, one crisis at a time. And remember, this, too, shall pass.

# Chapter 9

*When Is Enough Too Much?*

*—Your Mother*

*Y*ou may reach the point where you've had enough. I've been there many times. Life with someone who has bipolar disorder can become more of a challenge than you are willing to accept. Maybe the bipolar in your life won't take medication as prescribed, won't (or can't?) control a raging temper. It feels as if there are no more good times between the bad times.

Back up, slow down, breathe deep and reconsider. People with other diseases and disorders can be equally frustrating to live with. A loved one with any terminal illness, any ongoing condition like diabetes, asthma, Parkinson's disease, Cushing's disease, arthritis, lupus and many others would also cause changes in the personality of the person you fell in love with. Would you abandon a person because he or she had the type of diabetes that eventually causes blindness? Or Parkinson's that takes away voluntary muscle movements and sends a loved one thrashing and jerking at odd times? What about advanced cancer, when the patient has to be doped up until their brain can't function clearly? Would you leave someone you love over diseases like those?

If those or other illnesses caused or precipitated any type of abuse, then yes, you should and hopefully would leave. Otherwise, "in sickness and in health" is a good phrase to consider. Whether the bipolar person in your life is a good friend, relative, child or spouse, that person is in your life for a reason. Is that reason an accident of birth or because you think he or she is wonderful and exciting when in a mildly manic cycle.

If it is your child, help them grow as long as it is helpful. You cannot force a child who has reached adulthood into anything, whether it is in that child's best interest or not. You may have to stop helping in the same way, but you don't have to abandon or stop loving him or her. The same goes for other relatives.

If we're talking about a friend, spouse or significant other, did you at one time have great talks, go wonderful places? Laugh and cry together? Did that person ever come through for you? Or demonstrate genuine caring? You don't have to be married to decide on an "in sickness or in health" relationship.

Of course, there may come a time when you are getting so emotionally and physically drained that your health is endangered. You may have spent all you had and all you could borrow or charge trying to help. Hospitals and psychiatrists cost a lot of dollars, and many insurance policies cover a much smaller percent of expenses for psychiatric treatment than for other medical costs. So how much is too much?

Only you can decide.

I would never ask anyone else to go through what I've been through. If you are merely starting to date someone who is bipolar, my first advice would be, "Run!" But if you did that, you'd miss the strangest, wildest, most wonderful, most awful, scariest roller-coaster ride in the world.

If you're already in a relationship or marriage, you know about the good stuff and wonder where it goes from time to time. Who is this stranger in your life? In your bed? Is it enough to share a house when depression shuts down conversation? Or your phone calls aren't returned? Or when statements made in anger are hurtful? Yes, but only if you understand that whatever is going on in the bipolar's head probably has no bearing on what you've done or who you are. Listen, just to be sure, though. We're not always right and we're certainly not always angels.

Separating me from Bob's actions, and sometimes his accusations, has saved me from sinking into a depression of my own. If I'd stay tied to his fluctuating opinion of me, I'd never have been able to know who I am and what I like or don't like. He always loves me. He likes me most of the time. When he's depressed, he sometimes blames me for whatever he feels is wrong in his life. When he's manic, I'm the most beautiful, sexy woman of all time.

So, who am I, really? I'm an ordinary wife, mother, ex-legal secretary, mystery author, aunt, sister, grandmother, associate and friend. I fill many roles with many people. I am separate from him, though we have been together for a long time. When he hurts, I hurt. I hurt for him. I hurt for me. Neither of us wants the pain of illness clouding our thoughts and actions. It is there. It is always there. Is it too much? Have I had enough? Not today.

I realize not everyone feels as I do, nor is every person with bipolar disorder willing to work as hard for his or her own mental health as Bob is.

I have made decisions to stay after much prayer and meditation, much observation and experience. You will have to make your own decision on when enough is too much.

I do have several guidelines I use. One of the main criteria is my evaluation of the danger involved. I like my body. It serves me as best it can. I will not allow anyone to damage it. Physical violence, as I have stated several times throughout this book, must not be tolerated under any circumstances. It does not matter how much I love him. It does not matter how sorry he would be afterward. That is unacceptable.

The only time he ever threatened to beat the **** out of me "if I ever talked to him like that again," he was across the room. He stomped off to his den. I ran to our bedroom and threw a few things into a suitcase. I was out of there in less than five minutes.

Through phone calls and, finally, a meeting, we agreed we needed to see a counselor. We stayed in therapy until we were both satisfied that it would never happen again. It hasn't, and that was over five years ago.

During the time I was gone, I never doubted I loved him, nor did I doubt his love for me. I did know that unless something changed, I could never again live with him. I have no desire to live with him unless I am able to trust that I am in no physical danger. Today, I have that trust completely.

I'm grateful he was willing to change, to go to therapy, to talk to Dr. Hauser about his medication, and to do whatever else it took to get us back to our version of normal. We both had to work at it. Life is, truly, a series of overcoming obstacles.

Another way I measure the current status is with this question: Does the good still outweigh the bad? When it doesn't, I promise myself to give our relationship one more week before I make any permanent decision. For all these years, it has always changed before the week is up.

My strict rules are the three A's: abuse, addiction and affair. I've already covered abuse, but untreated addiction to alcohol and/or drugs can cause the other two A's.

If drug addiction or alcoholism is a problem, there is so much help available. Alcoholics Anonymous and Alanon Family Groups[4] (for family and friends of anyone with a drinking problem, and Narcotics Anonymous[5] have no dues or fees, so cost can't be an excuse for a bipolar not seeking help.

It is not necessary to go through a treatment center or hospital to become a member of either organization. However, most health insurance policies cover part of the cost if a treatment facility is preferred or required for detoxification.

If the bipolar refuses to get help with an alcohol or drug problem, by all means go to Alanon Family Groups, an organization of friends and families of alcoholics. Their meetings will help you understand your role in the relationship and how to change it. If one of you doesn't change, everything will continue to get worse.

The last measure of whether I am willing to stay in this marriage is simple. As long as Bob is willing to take part in the maintenance of his own mental health, I'll stay. I don't think I could stay if he quit taking his medication, quit exercising, quit trying to help others or overtly refused to accept treatment for his illness. If that should happen, I'd still check

---

4  If you cannot find a listing in your local telephone book, the number for locating an Alanon meeting near you is 1-800-344-2666.

5  Narcotics Anonymous can be contacted by calling 1-800-896-8896.

out all the other guidelines before I made a decision to leave.

Some few manic-depressives seem able to control their severe mood swings with alternative medicine (diet, meditation, herbs, massage therapy and such). I have no objection to anything that works. If the bipolar is trying, it counts.

If he or she is not trying, I couldn't stick around and wait for the end. I know I could not sit passively by and watch an alcoholic or addict drink and drug himself to death, either. For Bob to quit taking his medication would amount to an alcoholic returning to the bottle, an addict returning to drugs. That is when too much would be enough for me.

As long as any manic-depressive is trying, I believe that person should be supported, encouraged and loved.

I'll admit that some days I wonder if I've made the right choice. Staying is often not easy, but it is always what I want to do. Sometimes I stay only one day at a time. Most days I know it is a lifetime commitment.

If you continue to love that bipolar in your life, I can promise you this: Your life will be a lot of things, but it will never be dull.

In the meantime, look to your own mental, physical and spiritual health. Get to know what services are available for you in your area. Here are some of the things I do to take care of me so I can be supportive of him:

- Read uplifting literature. Whether spiritual, like the Bible or *Sermon on the Mount* by Emmet Fox, or a novel of courage and honor, or a magazine article sharing one person's success, I try to read something elevating every day.

- Exercise your brain. Learn something. I have no desire to be a financial consultant, but I took a licensing course to stretch my mind and to learn new, conservative ways to plan for our future financial independence. I had to study. I believe learning delays aging and increases confidence. I've also gone back to college and taken Speech, something that didn't appeal to me during my earlier college experience.

- Do something. Plant a garden even if it is only in old coffee cans. Clean out a closet. Paint a T-shirt. Go to a movie with a friend. Make a new friend. Write a poem. Go to the zoo. Go where the tourists in your area go. Find a shut-in to visit.

I have tried all these and more. When I am concentrating on trying to do something, it takes my focus off Bob. Even though I need to be aware of his moods, I do not need to have his mental health at the center of my thoughts.

To be of maximum help to him, I must find and develop my talents, my friends, and my relationship with God. My carrying the burden of Bob is not beneficial to either of us. Walking beside him, holding his hand from time to time, is beneficial to both of us.

Do anything and everything, but don't let the manic-depressive in your life be your excuse for doing nothing you enjoy.

# Chapter 10

*Life is too critical to take seriously*

*—Unknown.*

*T*here are five recognized senses: sight, hearing, touch, smell and taste. Then there's common sense, a sixth sense (intuition), and best of all, a sense of humor. The latter seems necessary for mental and physical health.

When I was a child, I took myself and everything in life very seriously. It all seemed so extremely important. It is, but it doesn't have to be a glum struggle.

Lighten up! No matter what happens, with or without you, the world will go on. It's great to stop and smell the roses, but without laughter, even the roses cease to look beautiful.

Cheerfulness, a glad heart, the happiness we search for can often be found in a good laugh. A good laugh is one that makes everyone feel better. If the laughter is at someone's expense, maybe it's not such a good laugh, after all.

I love word-play jokes like the one about a bear who walks into a saloon and orders a sandwich. He eats the sandwich, then goes over to the piano player and shoots him dead. As he leaves the saloon, the bartender, afraid of making the bear mad, cautiously asks, "Would you mind telling me why you shot my piano player?" The bear says, "It's in dictionary. Look it up." The bartender pulls down his Webster's and turns to the B's. Sure 'nuff, there it is. *Bear: noun; eats shoots and leaves.*

It is the unexpected twist that makes us laugh. Life is full of them. Whenever I do something silly or stupid, I confess to Bob, with a big build-up, that he married nut. By the time I get to the punch line, he and I are both laughing. It feels so good, too.

If you get upset over my using the word *nut*, you may be taking life 'way too seriously. In our house, we use words like crazy, nuts, insane, looney bin, Ha-ha or Banana Hilton, jitter joint, nutward, etc., without taking offense. They are words that deflect the fear of our potential future. We also refer to me as Gimpy or the cripple or just plain Crip.

I find that hearing the truth, even in such crass and insensitive terms, helps me deal with it as a natural part of my life. We don't try to hide the truth by not using "those words."

You probably don't have any trouble with someone calling you a blond or brunette or redhead, regardless of the color of your roots. It is what shows that elicits the choice of words. Your hair color is not all of you, but it is part of you. So? Why the big deal about my calling Bob a nutcase? Or calling myself a cripple?

Once, before my last surgery when I still had to wear a leg brace, I was in the grocery store shopping. A boy of about three or four openly stared at my shiny metal. His mother jerked him away, admonishing him in a loud whisper, "Don't stare. It's not nice." The boy, still wide-eyed, looked up at her, then pointed at my leg. "But, Mommy, I think it's bionic!"

I chuckled all the way home.

I had very little sense of humor when Bob and I married. I give him most of the credit for teaching me to laugh at myself and with others.

He has been told by more than one person that he has a warped sense of humor. Is there any other kind? Humor is a warped way of looking at life. It is seeing the ridiculous in the serious, the funny in the tragic.

While Bob was a patient on the psychiatric floor of Memorial Hospital, he called home and announced, "I'm the only rookie nut up here." Unfortunately, it was true.

He had asked one man why he had been hospitalized. He said, "My wife left me so I quit taking my medicine."

Bob asked, "Why? Did she take it with her?"

The man saw no humor in the question, but because all the other patients were return engagements, Bob set about to find out why. He discovered that every single one of the re-runs had stopped taking their prescribed pills—then wondered why they'd gotten sick again. Maybe that's why he's so medication compliant.

Whenever Bob does something silly, friends often tease him with, "Are you taking your meds?"

One of his comebacks is, "Yeah, and you ought to be glad I am."

I developed my sense of humor by listening, reading and observing. The world is really a very funny place. I also had the help of an old curmudgeon who often said, "Count yourself, you ain't so many."

It was hard to take myself so seriously after his knowing wink and smile. He had a way of letting me know that in the grand scheme of life, I am not any more or any less than anyone, but that I am, after all, only one. I'd laugh with him and say, "Guess I'm getting a little carried away with my own importance and my little problems."

Some of my problems are very real, very serious. Taking them seriously doesn't make them any more of a problem. Taking them lightly doesn't make them any lighter. Getting them into perspective, knowing that I can't take care of tomorrow's problems until they become today's makes today look pretty darned good.

Today, I have to laugh at some of the antics I've pulled, trying to look like I knew what I was doing. In the law office where I worked for several years, I made every mistake possible. I filed cases in the wrong court, hung up on a judge, and drank all the lawyer's Diet Cokes. When I first went to work for him, he proclaimed, "Anything you mess up, I can fix." I doubt if he told my successor that.

A lot of life is a location joke. You or someone else tries to tell a funny experience and no one laughs. The storyteller ends with, "Guess you had to be there."

To see the humor in life, you have to be there, taking part in life. Part of being there is listening, observing and staying in the now. You can't jump to the punch line and expect to get the joke.

When I'm frustrated and frantically trying to get a job done, I can see myself as Lucy on the assembly line, and I have take a laugh break.

When you really think about it, that was a sad scene. Here was a woman trying to do a job that she couldn't possibly do. The belt kept moving faster and faster. How frustrating! How sad. Yet, it is one of the funniest, most memorable scenes in her career.

Watch yourself sometime when you're trying to do something difficult. Would someone else see the humor in it? Then you can, too.

Listen to others and to yourself. Sometimes we say the silliest things. We reverse beginning sounds and come out with some real doozies. Instead of being embarrassed and stuttering on, try laughing at yourself. Everyone stumbles over words at some time or other. I've done it from the podium to a room full of students.

The same thing goes for when your brain goes into NUM LOCK and you can't remember you own phone number. Others will laugh with you if you don't take yourself too seriously.

When we watch a comedian perform, we expect to laugh, we want to laugh. If the show is really good, we can't *not laugh* no matter what mood we were in when the show began.

I'm not pretending that loving a manic-depressive is a laughing matter, but without the laughter, you can become so glum that your manic-depressive won't want to be around you. Then who is the nutcase?

If your sense of humor is really low, start at the bottom. Watch cartoons. Read a funny book. But most of all, quit taking yourself and your problems so seriously. We've all got problems. Yours may be unique to you, but you are not that unique.

In upgrading my sense of humor, I keep a notebook of funny or bizarre things that happen each day. Only one incident is recorded. This exercise keeps me watching for the humor in my life.

I also have a few friends I can call and say, "You'll never believe what I did today." Then I proceed to tell them about setting the coffeepot in the refrigerator and waiting for it to drip.

Stick with me and you can be funny, too.

# Chapter 11

*But let there be spaces in your togetherness, and let the winds of the heavens dance between you*
*—Kahlil Gibran.*

*M*utual recovery. Is it possible? If so, what does it mean?

What it doesn't mean is that a manic-depressive recovers from the brain disease like he or she would from a broken leg or bacterial infection. It doesn't mean that you quit feeling that panic-acid in the pit of your stomach from time to time, wondering if the bipolar is okay.

No one in life is exempt from life. Ups and downs are part of life. It is a miracle that any of us can live in a dwelling with another of us even in the best of circumstances. We each know what we want. We each have a firm idea of how what we want should be delivered. It never happens that way. We become disillusioned. We grouse at each other. We blame each other. And where does it get us? Separated.

Even if we are not physically separated, the wall between us grows until it can become insurmountable.

If we allow that to happen, it is very difficult for either one of us to give in to the other. This is where the concept of giving in to the relationship is vital.

Debbie, a woman I've shared with on many occasions, confessed she hated to admit she was wrong even when she knows she is. I believe this is a universal feeling during any argument. Whether right or wrong, no one likes to feel forced to surrender. It doesn't make any difference if we're surrendering an opinion, a perception or an idea. If we admit the other person is right, it means we are automatically wrong.

As Debbie put it, "Why do I always have to be the one who says I'm sorry? Sometimes I'm not, but if I don't apologize, he won't talk to me."

I explained that to me an apology or an admission of wrongdoing or guilt is not something anyone wants to offer. If I know I'm wrong, guilty or being obstinate about a point, it is easier to 'fess up. If I don't think I'm wrong, I surrender to the relationship. I honestly want it to work. In order for it to work, one of us has to give in. I give in to the relationship, to the concept that we are better off together than alone. I also believe strongly that who is wrong and who is right is unimportant. I can be technically right, but I am wrong if I cling to the idea that Bob has to understand that I am right. He doesn't. Clinging to that idea can keep us separated to the gates of Divorce Court.

On the other hand, separation is not always a bad thing. Some separation is necessary. No matter how much I love Bob, no matter how much I love my children, no matter how much they love me, they don't want me around twenty-four hours a day every day.

Best friends don't need to be together constantly, either.

To maintain any relationship, it is necessary for each member of the relationship to have some time alone and some time with other people. When you love a bipolar, that can get tricky.

Some bipolars insist their spouse or significant other be, at all times, where they can be reached. Whether this stems from fear of depression or fear of abandonment or a desire to control, it is important to the bipolar. In those cases, a cell phone can be one solution.

Some bipolars, especially in a manic state, even a mild one, may work long hours and sleep little. They may stay gone and be outraged that you'd dare ask where they've been. Does it matter?

The constants seems to be that they don't want anyone clinging to them, don't want anyone telling them what to do, and don't want to be alone even when they are telling you to go away. It doesn't take a mind reader to see what the problem is. They don't understand what they want any better than you do.

Wanting to be independent may make you resent having to be available. Independence is highly prized these days. I strongly agree with the concept, but being independent or being dependent is not the problem. Today, I am independent because I can choose to love Bob, and I choose to live with him.

I never felt more committed to our relationship until I could stay in my marriage because I wanted to, not because I had to. I could earn a living; I could take care of myself; I could live alone. Knowing I could make it freed me to stay.

I am not an extremely organized person. In fact, I'm more disorganized than most. I do try to take life as it comes. I try to have food in the house. I know we're going to want to eat again. I try to pay bills on time because I suspect we're going to want the lights and water to stay functional. I do not try to guess what Bob wants. I ask.

I know that sounds simple. I know I don't always get a straight answer, but it sure beats my crystal ball.

We try to be honest with each other. If I ask him if he wants me to go with him to the doctor and he says, "No," I don't go. If I want him to go shopping with me, I'd better tell him straight out, "I'd like for you to go shopping with me." If I ask, "Would you like to go with me?" he will most likely decline. After an invitation like that, I have no excuse for acting as if my feelings are hurt.

Three rules I try to follow are:

1. Don't give options unless they are requested.

2. Don't harp on anything that has already been decided.

3. Don't nag about anything that hasn't been done exactly to your specifications.

Options allow for answers you don't want. Be specific. If you don't get the answer you're fishing for, don't whine. You gave the options. Next time, be more direct. As much as we think we can read another's mind, we also tend to expect them to read ours. We can't read theirs; they can't read ours. I try not to fall into the trap of "If he'd paid attention, he'd know I would rather have a new red blouse than another bathrobe." How can he possibly know if I haven't told him what I want?

Nagging can become a way of life. If the garbage isn't carried out even when you've agreed it is his chore, you nag. If towels or underwear don't make it to the hamper, you nag. If newspaper seems to be reproducing in the den, you nag. These are universal complaints and have nothing to do with bipolar illness. Nagging will never change the behavior of another person. This goes double for manic-depressives.

When I look at the complaints in the preceding paragraph, I wonder why any of us get bent out of shape over such minor annoyances. If the garbage spills over, will it really matter? If you pick up after him, will it make you any less loving? Or less of a person? If something is important to me, it makes sense that I take care of it

One of the exercises I use to keep our relationship functioning smoothly follows:

1. At the top of a sheet of paper or the first line on a page in your computer write: HE does...

2. Make a list of everything he does that ticks you off.

3. On another page, write: HE doesn't...

4. Make another list of everything he doesn't do that ticks you off.

5. Set the list aside for twenty-four hours.

6. At the top of the first page, place an "S" in front of HE.

7. Being as honest as possible, read the list slowly and see how much it fits.

8. Do the same with the second list.

You may be amazed.

I often complained to myself or others (if not to him), that he never came and found me to kiss me goodbye when he left the house. When I put that on my list and changed the "he" to "she," I had to admit I was equally guilty. Instead of complaining or nagging, I began to always kiss him goodbye. Within a few weeks, he was doing the same for me.

Once a decision is made to go somewhere or do something together, don't spend any time going over and over it. Indicating you don't like the decision and want to reopen the discussion is another way of saying you didn't get your way. Vacations, movies, restaurants will all be there the next time you're deciding.

There are some movies I like that he can't stand the thought of sitting through. That's when I take a neighbor, or a neighbor's kid or go alone. As for restaurants, if I want to eat at a restaurant he doesn't care for, I invite a friend to lunch.

Being together is more than doing things together.

If you want to learn about togetherness, remember what brought you together in the first place. Drag out some of the romance you left at the altar. A manic-depressive partner doesn't cease being the person you met and fell in love with, anymore than you quit being you. We all change. Sometimes the change is good; sometimes it isn't so good. If we didn't grow and change, we'd still be in diapers.

In spite of the changes, most of the basics are still there. Look for them. Remember you are two people who care about each other. One of you has bipolar disorder. It is an illness; it is not the person.

This point was clearly illustrated when Bob had to go back to the hospital because of his illness. He had done everything right: maintained his medication schedule, exercised and spent time with his support group. We have known from the beginning that lithium is a powerful and potentially toxic medication. He has always been careful to drink extra water on the days he jogs so that the lithium doesn't get concentrated from lack of body fluids. It never occurred to us that a case of vomiting and diarrhea would deplete his fluids and salts. Of course, we knew there was a danger of him becoming dehydrated, but since he couldn't hold anything on his stomach, he didn't take in enough fluid. He continued to take the lithium.

Within two days, he changed from just-a-virus sick to very seriously sick. His body jerked and shook as if he had palsy. His thoughts were jumbled; he couldn't focus on what he was trying to say; he shuffled and stumbled. He had severe panic attacks.

I rushed him to the emergency room. The doctor there had his lithium blood level checked. It was extremely high. He was admitted to the hospital and medicated to keep him calm. By the third day off the lithium, his blood levels had dropped to acceptable levels. He wasn't responding to the drop as the doctor had expected. An Electroencephalograph (EEG) was scheduled to determine if there was any brainwave disturbance. By the time for the test, he'd made exceptional progress and was allowed to go home.

Eventually, everything straightened out, and he was back to his wonderful self.

During that episode, he said I didn't love him and had him locked up because I wanted a vacation. He got out his pistol and wanted to shoot himself because "it" wouldn't leave him alone. He hallucinated and cried, saying it was my fault. He looked as if he aged twenty or thirty years. His shoulders drooped, his eyes looked watery and his mumbling became unintelligible.

It was very scary to watch a strong man turn into a shuffling, irrational man I did not recognize or know. Throughout the ordeal, I knew and trusted that the awful things he said were the illness talking, not him. I spent several hours each day holding him, knowing he was very sick, not knowing if he would recover.

It all seemed so unfair, but then only some blondes and occasionally the weather are fair. No one ever promised life would be fair. I had to remember we were dealing with disease. Cancer isn't fair. Diabetes isn't fair. It did seem that by doing everything he was told would produce the desired results. It didn't. It wasn't fair. We survived; we drew closer. We won!

And so can you.

# Chapter 12

*So you're not a joiner, join anyway*

—Me.

No matter how independent we want to be, we need people. For thousands of years people have congregated in tribes, villages, towns and cities. In our past, extended families lived together or at least very close by. We learned from each other; we learned to live with each other. The generations weren't separated.

In today's mobile society we don't have the close-knit families that once dominated our culture. Most of us live more than a hundred miles from our family of origin. Those of us who do live in close proximity to the grandparents and great-grandparents of our children seldom trust our elders to guide us through life's rough spots. We tend to believe we can learn only from personal experience. We think life is a "do by self" project, as one of my sisters used to demand.

Living with or loving someone who has bipolar disorder further tends to isolate us. Our families don't understand why we stay. They have a variety of ideas and misconceptions about what we should and shouldn't do. We may resent their suggestions, in spite of their good intentions. Then we feel guilty for our feelings. Or we feel justified in our resentments.

We need people who understand what we're going through, people who have been there, or are there and can show us how they do it without self-pity.

It is only the more intelligent of the species that learn from the mistakes of others and grow emotionally by following the examples of others. In this age of support groups, it is difficult not to find one that addresses problems similar to yours. Our problems don't have to be identical, but our solutions do. If I have a broken leg, set the bone and keep it immobile for about six weeks, it will heal. If you have a broken leg and follow the same procedure, you will get the same results.

This healing pattern works for emotional and spiritual maladies, too. If I do what others in my group have done, I will get the results they got. In our exchange of solutions, it is important that we see people who have been living with difficult circumstances for a long time and who seem to be coping. If we all start from the same spot, we could make progress, but it would be through trial and error instead of shared experience.

Bob and I are fortunate to live in Houston, where there are several DMDA meetings a week. We also have a network of support through a Fellowship that is spiritual in nature, practical in application.

I believe that a spiritual solution to living problems, no matter how large the problems, is the only solution. Whether you practice a religion or not is immaterial. The important concept is to develop spiritually.

Any exploration into methods of meditation can be a beginning. I have used a combination of ideologies and religions during the past years and come up with a method and literature that supports my endeavors. If you are involved in a church or synagogue, you will want to use your religion as a base. No matter where you start, you still need to find a group of people heading in the same direction you want to go.

God, as I understand Him, often works through people. By getting involved with learning from and helping others, I get out of God's way and give Him the opportunity to guide me, bless me, and soothe my troubled thoughts.

In my morning meditation I ask Him to direct my thinking and my actions. Then I call two people from my group, one who is new to the group and one who was there when I showed up.

If there is no established DMDA group in your area, please contact one of the national organizations listed at the end of this chapter. Their headquarters may be able to direct you to a group close enough that the drive would be worth it, or they may help you begin a group along their guidelines for your neck of the woods.

Other possibilities include attending any group function on a regular basis. The possibilities are wide open: study groups, Bible or church groups, service organizations such as Rotary or Kiwanas, etc. Whatever you select, get involved. Get to know the others and let them know you. Sharing any burden lightens the load for everyone.

If you are afraid to talk about being married to a mental patient, please spend some time writing out your fears. Seeing them in black and white will help get them into perspective. Generally, our fears are unfounded or extremely self-centered. By self-centered, I mean that we are centering in on ourselves and what we suspect others are thinking of us. The truth is that most of the time, others are not thinking of us at all. They are caught up in their own lives, sometimes wondering what we think of them.

It is up to folks like you and me to change the world's opinion of mental patients. One organization monitors news media and calls them to task if they present anything that lumps all mental illnesses into one crazy pile. Like physical illnesses, mental illnesses range from "hangnail" to "heart attack" in severity, and from dangerous to docile in reactions. To state that a criminal perpetrator has a history of mental illness is tantamount to claiming another criminal has a history of diabetes. That information isn't pertinent to a news story because diabetes does not influence behavior. To lump all mental patients into the category of "dangerous" does untold damage to the mentally ill. The stigma is slowly being removed but it is so very slowly.

According to an article in *The Dallas Morning News* in 1996, by Tom Siegfried and Sue Goetinck, mental patients are no more violent than people in general. The incidence of elevated risk of violence equals the difference in tendencies between men and women, or teenagers and adults.

The authors quote Bruce Link, a psychiatric epidemiologist at the Columbia University School of Public Health in New York, who said, "If you want to protect yourself from violence, you would do just as well to avoid men and teenagers as you would to avoid people with mental illness."

Changing the public image of mental patients, or people with neurobiological disorders, through education, advocacy, support, and research is one of the goals of The Alliance for the Mentally Ill/Friends and Advocates of the Mentally Ill (AMI/FAM). For more information on how to become a member of the organization and receive their newsletter, contact AMI/FAM, 432 Park Avenue South, New York, NY 10016.

# Resources

National headquarters for other organizations and support groups may be reached by contacting them at the addresses listed below:

**National Institute of Mental Health**
Public Inquiries, Room 7C-02
5600 Fishers Lane
Rockville, MD 20857

**National Depressive & Manic Depressive Association**
730 Franklin Street, Suite 501
Chicago, IL 60610
Phone: (800) 826-3632

**National Alliance for the Mentally Ill**
2101 Wilson Boulevard, Suite 302
Arlington, VA 22201
Phone :(800) 950-NAMI (6264)

**National Foundation for Depressive Illness**
P O Box 2257
New York, NY 10016
Phone: (800) 248-4344

**National Mental Health Association**
1201 Prince Street
Alexandria, VA 22314-2971
Phone: (703) 684-7722

Please take advantage of the information available through these organizations and support groups. If you don't feel what I call a "heart tug" at one of the meetings, try another. Give yourself a chance to receive the help offered. I strongly suggest you try attending regularly for at least three months. It takes that long for most people to feel at home on a job, in a school or in a church. You deserve at least the same consideration from yourself, for yourself.

While you are adapting to a support group, try the suggested exercises in this book. They have helped me and many other people who love, and, yes, sometimes hate, a manic-depressive. No matter how hopeless you feel, there is more to life that walking on eggshells. There is, after all, a great sense of freedom available to you. Grab it, and go forward with God's blessing on you, and live your life while loving that manic-depressive.

The Beginning...